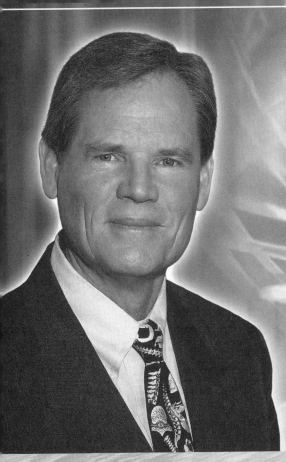

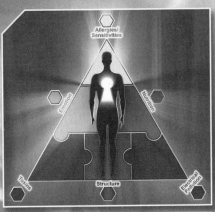

Dr. John Brimhall
&
Dr. Brett Brimhall

SOLVING THE HEALTH PUZZLE
— WITH —
THE 6 STEPS TO WELLNESS

Dr. John Brimhall
BESTSELLING INTERNATIONAL AUTHOR, LECTURER AND INVENTOR

SOLVING THE HEALTH PUZZLE
——— WITH ———
THE 6 STEPS TO WELLNESS

Copyright © 2007 **by Dr. John Brimhall &**
Dr. Brett Brimhall
Publisher **e2iBooks**
Cover Design & Layout **e2iBooks**
Edited by **Janell DeWitt**

For information, write to: **e2iBooks**
1800 Pembrooke Drive 3rd Floor
Orlando, FL 32810

The **e2iBooks** name and logo are registered trademarks of **e2iBooks**

Printed in the United States of America

Second edition **e2iBooks** printing: November 2007
First edition **e2iBooks** printing: January 2006

Library of Congress Cataloging-in-Publication Data

Brimhall, John (John Wayne), 1947-
Solving The Health Puzzle With The 6 Steps To Wellness / John
Brimhall and Brett Brimhall. -- 1st ed.
p. cm.
ISBN 978-1-60221-993-9 (pbk. : alk. paper)
1. Health. 2. Medicine, Preventive. 3. Holistic medicine. 4. Self-care,
Health. I. Brimhall, Brett, 1974- II. Title.
RA776.B772 2007
613--dc22
2007026679

Solving the Health Puzzle with the 6 Steps to Wellness is not intended as a substi-
tute for the advice and/or medical care of the reader's physician, nor is it meant to
discourage or dissuade the reader from the advice of his or her physician. Readers
should regularly consult with a physician in matters relating to his/her health, especially with symptoms that may require diagnosis. If the reader has any questions
concerning the information presented in this book, or its application to his or her
particular medical profile, or if the reader has unusual medical or nutritional needs
or constraints that may conflict with the advice of this book, he or she should
consult his or her physician. The reader should not stop prescription medications
without the advice and guidance of his or her personal physician.

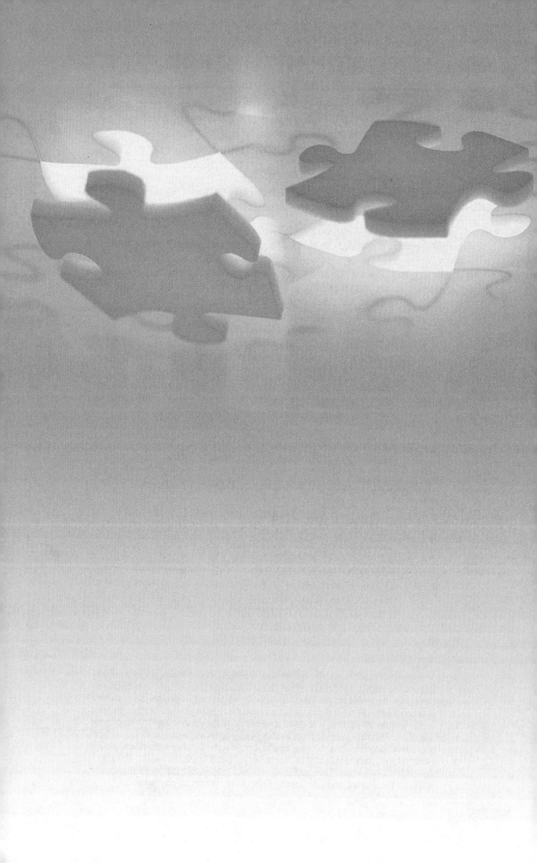

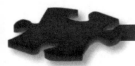

TABLE OF CONTENTS

STEP 2

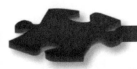

WHAT PATIENTS AND DOCTORS ARE SAYING ABOUT SOLVING THE HEALTH PUZZLE WITH THE SIX STEPS TO WELLNESS

Autoimmune Disease

Dear Dr. Brimhall,

Words cannot adequately express the thanks and appreciation I feel for what you have done for me, but knowing the dedication you have in helping people to heal, perhaps my story will help others.

In 1998, I went to Mayo Clinic in Minnesota and was diagnosed with an "unspecified autoimmune disease." This, my doctor explained, was why I was suffering with flu-like symptoms, arthritic pain in all my joints and lack of energy. He told me the treatment for autoimmune disease would not be wise at that time because the treatment was far worse than the disease. I asked if there was anything I could do to make things better, and he suggested rest, diet, exercise and to accept the fact that there would be days where I would feel like I had the flu all over my body. I left feeling like this was my "lot in life" and that I needed to make the most of it. Within a year, my symptoms had increased in frequency and intensity and my local rheumatologist, who had taken care of me for more than 15 years, diagnosed me with lupus. He explained that, at any time, my autoimmune disease could attack my kidneys, lungs, heart or brain. He immediately prescribed cortisone and said he would consider other medications for me as well. I filled the prescription and took it with me on an extended summer vacation but was concerned about taking the pills.

That summer I tried my best to "make memories" with my husband because I could see the deterioration of my health. We had altered our lives around my health and had even cancelled the building of our yacht.

By the first of September 2000, I was getting worse and my local chiropractor felt I needed a far more aggressive approach. He said if he were in my position, he would go to the Brimhall Clinic. My husband insisted that I call the clinic. I was told the soonest they could schedule an appointment for me was in January 2001. That was more than 3 months away!

Meanwhile, my rheumatologist scheduled a CAT scan of my brain. The result of having that scan created an unbelievable reaction. Not only did it intensify my symptoms, it made me totally weak. If I went near power lines, the computer, or fluorescent lights, I got worse. (I later learned some medical doctors do not suggest that a patient in a heightened autoimmune state have such a scan because there is evidence of adverse reactions.) I had reached such a low point - I was unable to drive, work in my home, and most of my days were spent in agony. I felt the medical arena had nothing to offer me but tests that would make me worse and medicine that would eventually kill me.

At my husband's insistence, I called the Brimhall Clinic and asked to personally speak to Dr. John Brimhall. When he returned my call, I told him my history and that I truly didn't feel I would be alive if I didn't get in before my January appointment. He said he felt he could help me and would see what he could do to get my appointment moved up. The next day his office called with an appointment for October 30th. My body was worn out, and my state of mind was not hopeful. I felt I had to go to the Brimhall Clinic at least for my husband's peace of mind.

The first day we arrived I felt as if I was in an emergency room. Dr. Brimhall and his fantastic team began work on me. They helped me to unload all types of toxins from heavy metals to emotional toxins and began to restore my electromagnetic field. By day two, I had renewed hope, and by day three, I felt energy I hadn't felt in months and months! I was still very sick; after all, I had been with this condition for years, and the mere fact that in three days I could have renewed energy was miraculous!

I was so thrilled with my progress I wanted to make up for lost time. I was ready to go to the Grand Canyon that weekend. Dr. Brimhall, in his wisdom, drew a chart for me explaining there would be peaks and valleys for a while. Of course, he was right. He explained the road to "Wellness" was not a destination but a journey. There were "tough" days, but my faith and trust in Dr. Brimhall and his techniques kept me dedicated, focused and on track to do what

16

was needed to restore my health. He had proven without doubt that I could be helped – it was up to me to stay the course.

It has all been well worth it – as I have my active lifestyle back. We were able to get back to boating extensively. When there was no hope – it was given! When there was no good health – it was restored!

Less than a year after my initial treatment with Dr. Brimhall, I returned to Mayo Clinic for an assessment of my autoimmune condition. My doctors were able to see a symptom-free patient with an ANA blood test in the normal range for the first time in years! My husband and I have continued to go to the Brimhall Clinic for annual checkups or "tune-ups" as my husband refers to them with Dr. Brett Brimhall. I have maintained my good health, I have taken my children there and have recommended the clinic to many friends. One of my medical doctor friends, after observing my restored health, was amazed and went to the clinic and found the treatments very beneficial. It has been such a joy to see the help my children and friends have received.

We are so very thankful for the dedication and work of the Brimhall System of Wellness.

— Judie B.

The Standard American Diet

My health challenge began three years ago when an already depleted body, caused by 55 years of the standard American diet and "normal" life stresses, contracted several bouts of flu while on a foreign work assignment. Medical doctors there prescribed normal pain and fever reducers, and I got on with my work and life (I thought!). These bouts left me with chronic diarrhea, nagging kidney pains, sharp gall bladder/liver pains and intestinal pains. By the end of my six-month assignment, I was beginning to lose weight and was suffering from fatigue. When I returned to the States, I checked in with my primary care physician, who thought I might have contracted a parasitic infection and immediately put me on an antibiotic therapy. It didn't get better! Over the next two years, I consulted with 18 different doctors who scheduled a total of five colonoscopies, four upper endoscopies, seven CT or MRI scans, and multiple blood, urine and stool studies at a cost of over $30,000 to my insurance company. Finally, after visiting the Mayo Clinic in Rochester, Minnesota, I was diagnosed with Irritable Bowel Syndrome and told there was no cure. I started investigating alternative medicine channels. It was at this time that Dr. John Brimhall's Wellness Center was recommended by my local chiropractor. Dr. Brett Brimhall treated me daily for two weeks with amazing results. I decided to return to the Brimhall Wellness Center for whatever time it took to really get a state of wellness back. Now, at the end of this three-month program, I know the path to wellness. I now feel I have been given the skills to continue on the path of a lifetime of wellness.

— Frank T.

Depression

I hope my story will help whoever reads it. I was living a perfect life with happiness, joy and a love for the Lord like no other. But then my father was diagnosed with kidney cancer and passed away. I fell into a deep depression, which led to drugs and other disastrous things. My world went from joy to hell in a matter of weeks. I was living in an apartment with about five people. I was doing lots of cocaine and other things. I wasn't eating right. My body pretty much shut down. I could hardly stand up straight. I was having severe panic attacks and I was very skinny. Finally I decided, with God's help, to walk away from hell on earth. That's when I came to Dr. Brimhall and Dr. Reed for help. They taught me how to get well again through nutrition, vitamin supplements, adjustments and positive, good thoughts. I believe that the Lord worked through both of those people.

— Tim B.

Stunted Growth

Dear Dr. John,

You will remember our little grandson, Tyler M., son of Ed and Marie M. from Ketchikan, Alaska. He was the 5-year-old who spoke like an adult but looked like a 3-year-old. Because of Marie's concern that Tyler was not growing normally (1/4 inch in the previous year), she brought him to you in early June of 1998. She asked that each of your staff treat Tyler, as we had told her that each of the doctors in your clinic had a special talent. So all of you will be pleased to know that since you treated him during June and they returned to Ketchikan, he has grown *1¼ inches* in the last three months. We want to thank you for all you have done for us, our children and our grandchildren who have been helped so much at the clinic.

— Kent C.

In Pain

I distrusted chiropractors. I thought they were quacks who cracked necks. At seventeen, I had had a bad experience with one in Tennessee. Fortunately, good friends introduced my husband and me to Dr. Brimhall. There I found a path to wholeness, peace of mind and relief from pain. I have proof that following the doctor's orders works. My chest no longer feels like something heavy is sitting on it. My neck isn't stiff, it's relaxed and flexible! Recently, while singing a hymn in church, my voice became clear and free for the first time in 10 years. A chronic pain in my right foot had kept me from walking comfortably for several years. Now my foot is as good as new! I no longer have to take anti-acid pills. I sleep all night long!

— Fay E.

Prostatitis & Depression

When I came to the clinic three months ago with severe prostatitis, my life was miserable. I considered suicide on more than one occasion. My feelings were all bottled up, and I felt very depressed. It was a battle most days just to get out of bed. After I left the clinic, everything changed. My depression is over. Suicide is the furthest thing from my mind. My symptoms have almost completely subsided. This is a huge accomplishment when you consider that I had seen some of the leading authorities on my illness, and none of them gave this kind of relief. I love life now, and I owe it all to the Brimhall Wellness Center.

— John V.T.

Brimhall Wellness Seminars

At the Las Vegas show last June, we heard Dr. John Brimhall for the first time. We were so impressed that we drove to his clinic for treatment. Since then, we have been back to see him on two occasions, driving over 2,000 miles from Jupiter, Florida, to Mesa, Arizona. He has proven to be an excellent doctor, very caring and truly dedicated to healing people.

— Francis E.N.

Regained the Use of an Arm

Dear Dr. Brimhall,

I want to thank you for the wonderful care you have given me. At our first meeting less than a year ago, I couldn't lift my left arm. I had been to several medical doctors and had no relief or improvement. Since receiving treatments at your clinic, I have regained about 85% use of my arm, and it's still improving. I have so much confidence in your ability and knowledge that I drive over 2,000 miles to your clinic, and it's really worth the trip.

— Ruth A. L.

Fibromyalgia

Dear Dr. Brimhall,

I was very pleased when I attended the recent Health Show in Las Vegas and finally found someone who can help my mother, Joyce S. of Clarkdale, Arizona, with her fibromyalgia (a chronic, widespread pain in muscles and soft tissues surrounding joints throughout the body). She has been in considerable pain for quite some time, and you certainly have given us hope.

— Dixie C.

One Doctor's Story

Dear Dr. Brimhall,

Thank you for everything you have done for my family and myself. I realize you have done a lot of extra things without charging me for them and have given me breaks on products and tapes, and although I do the same in my own practice every day, it is truly a blessing to be treated so kindly by another. The dual treatment mode with Mary Pat was something I will hold in my heart for all time. No matter what the future holds, I want you to know what a tremendous impact you have made on my life and my practice. Frankly, there is no way to convey my thanks in simple words – so I will attempt to do it in my stewardship of your teaching and creativity and spirit of giving in my life and in my practice.

— Reid T.

Arthritis, Fibromyalgia and Sinus Problems

To my friends at the Brimhall Wellness Center:

I came to Arizona from Pennsylvania 18 years ago, riddled with arthritis, fibromyalgia and sinus problems. My friend, Enid, begged me to try the Brimhall Wellness Center. She got me an appointment – and the rest is history! I can't explain what happened, but the change in me was hard to believe. Dr. Hansen told me I'd have my taste and smell again. Hah! I hadn't had any for years! I can taste now! I have a new life, and my prayers were answered. My heartfelt thanks to all the wonderful doctors and staff who gave me hope for a better life. At 77 years of age – it's a miracle!

— Kay W.

The Quality of Care

Dear Dr. Brimhall:

It is extremely difficult to express in words how I feel about my week of care in your wonderful haven of health. Every aspect of your office exudes with proficiency, compassion and an indescribable spirit and aura of oneness with the universe.

— Richard E. B.

A Baby With Difficulty Breathing

When my son Brett was 4 days old, he stopped breathing while I was nursing him. We dialed 911 ... and were flown by helicopter to Phoenix Children's Hospital. There we spent a horrible week when Brett was seen by five different kinds of pediatric specialists, including a pulmonologist, neurologist, cardiologist, gastroenterologist and an infectious disease specialist. He underwent four spinal taps, had several different kinds of X-rays and tests, including an MRI, and had blood drawn from his feet and head many times. None of the specialists could figure out what was wrong with him. So Brett came home at 10 days old yoked up to an apnea monitor and an oxygen tank on wheels. When Brett was 6½ weeks old, a friend told me about a holistic chiropractor she had been to the year before. She thought it wouldn't hurt for me to take Brett to see him. I had always been leery of chiropractors but felt like I would try anything. I took Brett to Dr. Brimhall the next day, and our lives changed immediately. I continued to take Brett back to Dr. Brimhall twice a week, and by the end of May his at-home oxygen test results showed levels at 98-99, so he could be taken off oxygen. Today he is almost 7 months old and is a healthy, active little boy who started crawling a week ago.

— Sarah S.

A Patient's Foreword

by Jon Keyworth
Former Denver Broncos Running Back

I played professional football for the Denver Broncos from 1974 to 1980. During my tenure, I experienced nine major surgeries between 1971 and 1980. When we're young we rarely if ever acknowledge the abuse we're imposing upon ourselves until it's too late.

I want to share with you an experience that literally changed my life. Hopefully, you'll be able to believe there is hope that you can become healed. What I am sharing with you is a tried, tested and proven healing system that works; and, its changing people's lives.

In 1976, two large screws were implanted into both shoulders to prevent the joints from dislocating. The surgery was successful and allowed me to continue playing. I retired from the Denver Broncos in 1981 at the young age of 31. From that time untill March of 2002, I was able to

22

function yet experienced continual pain. I was taking large doses of over-the-counter drugs three to four times a day, completely unaware of the damage I was doing to my liver and kidneys.

In March of 2002, something popped in my left shoulder. The excruciating pain threw me directly on the floor. I stood up and looked in the mirror and noticed that a deep gap existed between the top of my left shoulder and my left bicep muscle. It looked like the left bicep muscle had just curled up inside my arm.

I immediately made an appointment with the top athletic orthopedic surgeons in the country. After a simple examination they informed me that I had torn the bicipetous muscle. This muscle connects the bicep muscle to the top of the shoulder rendering my left arm completely useless.

The doctors made it very clear that there was nothing they could surgically do to attach the torn muscle. The only recommendation offered was to give me an experimental shoulder replacement using pig muscle. They wanted to give me Vioxx that just killed six people. My wife voiced her objections and they said it was perfectly safe. Facing a serious dilemma, I decided not to proceed with the surgery based on my knowledge concerning the long-term adverse effects of joint replacement.

By September of 2002, the pain in my left shoulder had not decreased. The normal use of my left arm remained deficient. I continued with physical therapies but nothing worked. Discouraged, I was ready to proceed with the replacement surgery.

Then, a miracle took place. In this same month, my wife Claudia was attending a special health and wellness seminar sponsored by Dr. John Brimhall. I confess, I was very skeptical that any treatment other than surgery would fix my left shoulder, but I went to the seminar, I was desperate for a solution.

What I found and experienced at that seminar was incredible. Dr. David Lee, one of Dr. Brimhall's top certified practitioners, took me aside, listened and then began not only to treat me, but took the time to educate me about what he was doing and why. He taught me that every procedure, process, and technique he was using to treat my shoulder was predicated upon sound, proven scientific principles. The techniques and principles Dr. Lee used involved new methods and discoveries of light and energy frequency healing, and many other non-invasive, non-toxic natural healing processes. To make a long story short, after 45 minutes, I was able to raise and use my arm with full mobility and without pain for the first time in six months. I cannot explain what Dr. Lee did to fix my shoulder - but he did. Dr. Lee stated that he was able to turn the power on within my shoulder. I was able to play golf two days later and carry-on a normal life with a fully functioning arm. Every now and then my shoulder becomes sore and I experience some minor pain. With occasional inexpensive treatments I'm able to function normally in my everyday activities. I'm also gaining new strength in both arms and shoulders.

After experiencing what to me was a miracle, I began to examine and explore the potential of Dr. Brimhall's 6 Step Protocol in helping many of my friends and family. I have come to learn that this healing procedure can help people who suffer from chronic pain, fatigue, asthma, diabetes, cancer, heart disease, chemical or nutritional imbalances, depression, arthritis, allergies, digestive disorders, and many other degenerative diseases. Dr. Brimhall and his certified practitioners do not treat these diseases, they treat people who suffer from these degenerative diseases.

We Americans sit and wonder why we pour trillions of dollars each year into our sick care system, and continue to have serious, unresolved, on-going health problems. We visit a doctor who spends only three to four minutes listening to us, and then almost without exception writes a prescription for a toxic drug that only treats the symptoms, not the cause of the problem.

My quest for knowledge has given me great hope. I've learned that thousands of people across our country are being treated by Brimhall practitioners using natural medicines, supplements and therapies. They are discovering the human body has the most powerful desire and ability to heal itself without expensive toxic drugs, therapies, or invasive surgical procedures.

I now know that if you are suffering from diseases of degeneration, depression, stress or other emotional or physical traumas—there is hope. Dr. Brimhall's trained practitioners can help set your body on the correct path to heal itself.

A Doctor's Foreword
By Don Colbert, MD

Over the course of my medical career, I've had the opportunity to study under some of the top nutritionists, acupuncturists, naturopaths, neurologists, biological dentists, alternative medical physicians and homeopaths in the world. And yet, despite the vast knowledge I gained, there always seemed to be some piece of the puzzle missing. While attending one of Dr. Brimhall's nutritional seminars eight years ago, I found that missing piece. Dr. Brimhall's *6 Steps To Wellness* finally put everything into perspective for me... providing a major "missing link" in the healing process.

What is so stimulating about this type of work is that non-invasive therapeutic devices are used in treating the patient, fulfilling the Hippocratic Oath that states "First do no harm." But non-invasive certainly doesn't mean non-effective. The *6 Steps To Wellness* can be used to address simple illnesses such as the common cold, yet can also help treat extremely serious diseases such as Lou Gehrig's Disease (ALS).

It has been an extreme honor and a pleasure to work with Dr. Brimhall in his effort to bring wellness to the world. I'm certain that patients and physicians alike will benefit from learning the 6 main interferences to healing and the *6 Steps To Wellness* taught in this book.

I truly believe that Dr. Brimhall is one of the most gifted physicians I have ever met.

A PhD's Foreward

Lynn Toohey, PhD

Every once in a very rare while, someone comes along who not only has the knowledge and ability to make a difference in people's lives, but can also TEACH it to others. Dr. John Brimhall is that person. Never before have I met anyone like Dr. John, who I can refer tough cases to, knowing with the utmost confidence that they will improve. His unique skills and comprehension of the complete picture, the "Total Wellness" approach, have helped more people than I could ever begin to count.

The protocol, while easy enough to use, incorporates various modalities that strengthen each other in a genuine, powerful, holistic approach to wellness. I can remember, years ago, being present at one of Dr. John's 3-day weekend seminars. I ran into one of the participants outside the lecture hall and asked, "Are you enjoying the seminar?" As her eyes welled up with emotion and the tears began to fall, she exclaimed, "He's changed my life; I can't believe it." That is how I describe the reaction to Dr. John's teaching - you can't describe it. You have to FEEL it. In my never-ending awe for how he can relate his holistic knowledge so that other people can experience it, I am elated that he now has chosen the form of a book to educate more people about this awesome protocol.

Even though my biggest connection to Dr. Brimhall has been nutritional, I recognize that it is only one piece of the puzzle – but he explains how that very important piece strengthens, and is strengthened by, other modalities such as energy work. Dr. Brimhall has the skills and the know-how to make it all work together, maximizing the potential for using quality nutrition to improve health and make a difference.

If you haven't experienced the protocol, or you have and want to refresh, read this book. But, be forewarned that you must be prepared for it to change your life!

ACKNOWLEDGEMENTS

We thank our parents, who spent their whole lives in the service of others and who taught their children the work ethic; our wives, who have always been by our sides, no matter the task or the hour; our children, who never stop teaching us; Dr. George Goodheart, the father of kinesiology; Dr. Paul and Marcia White, who are pioneers in pharmaceutical-grade nutrition for Nutri-West; Steven Shanks of Erchonia Medical with his contributions in low level laser therapy; Dr. Robert Fulford, who gave the percussor technique to mankind; Dr. James Oschman, who has given us the background for our understanding of "Energy Medicine;" Dr. Lynn Toohey, for generously providing great additions as a guest author; Dr. Sheldon Deal, as a teacher, author and practitioner who represents the many doctors we, Dr. John and Dr. Brett Brimhall, have studied under, lectured or taught with; and the thousands of patients that have shared their lives with us.

> *"The doctor of the future will give no medicine, but will treat his patients in the care of the human frame, in diet, and in the cause and prevention of disease."*
> — Thomas A. Edison

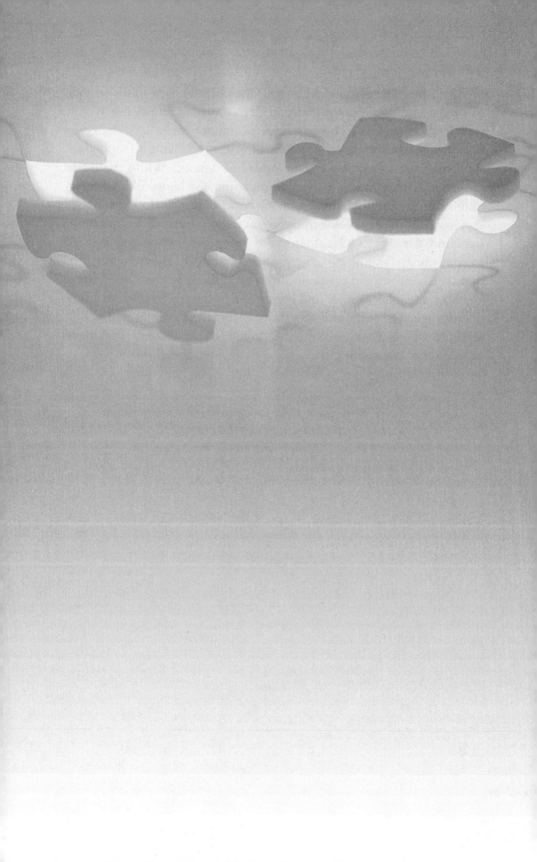

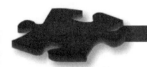

INTRODUCTION by Dr. John Brimhall

Everything happens for a reason, and plenty has happened to me. At age 18 I was in a car accident. A doctor said I had a whiplash. When I asked if I should see a chiropractor, he told me never; they might break my neck. So, of course I followed medical advice and took some pain relievers until I felt better.

I went relatively pain-free after a few weeks of medication, except for occasional stiffness in the back and neck. Two years later, at 20, I bent over and couldn't straighten up. My back went into a complete spasm, and my legs and feet went numb and tingly. I was bedridden in extreme pain. Conventional medicine offered me drugs or surgery, but wouldn't make any promises.

MY PERSONAL MIRACLE

On the advice of a cousin, I went to see a chiropractor and literally had to be carried into the office. The chiropractor x-rayed my spine and showed me that, in addition to other changes occurring, I had lost my cervical curve from the accident two years before.

He gave me my first spinal adjustment, and I felt a miracle take place. The feeling came back to my feet and legs, and the back spasms were gone almost instantly. The chiropractor explained that even though I was symptom-free after the spinal adjustment, my body needed corrective care and healing time to repair the damage that had been done.

He also suggested I become a chiropractor so I could do for others what chiropractic had done for me. The idea struck a chord. At the time I was in pre-dental studies, so a career shift required some serious, prayerful consideration.

Claudette, my wife of now over 37 years, was also in that accident with me during our dating years. She had been in one other accident three years earlier, which left her with constant headaches. As a wedding present, she received her first chiropractic adjustment, and her headaches vanished that very day. Our mutual healing experiences became the answer to our prayers.

It seemed that God had spoken to us. We felt we were intended to find out what natural healing and chiropractic were all about. So we changed our professional plans, knowing only that we had experienced miracles ourselves, and we were to serve others. A few months later, we were married, and on our way to Palmer College of Chiropractic. We've been on fire ever since, helping others just as we were helped ourselves. We learned early that the structure of the body controls its functions. As Dr. George Goodheart, the father of applied kinesiology said, "God will forgive you, but your nervous system will not."

WHITE MEDICINE MAN

Daniel David Palmer, the founder of modern chiropractic, once detected a pinched nerve in the back of a man who had gone deaf. By realigning the vertebrae, Harvey Lillard had his hearing restored.

Can miracles happen? We have found many times that they can. I became very successful with the structural adjustments used to enable the body to heal itself. In the first few months of practice, I adjusted Ida Chester, a Navajo Indian woman who was in a wheelchair. She had lost her bladder control and could no longer speak following an auto accident. After the first adjustment, her bladder control and speech returned. After her second adjustment she got out of the wheelchair. She began referring patients from all over the reservation.

Many of these patients didn't speak English and had no idea what we were doing, but they recognized that miracles were taking place. They began calling me the White Medicine Man.

The miracles continued. One woman had 14 years of migraines and tried relieving them with drugs, a hysterectomy and a vagus nerve surgery. Nothing worked. But after her first chiropractic adjustment, she never had a migraine again. We even saw people with diabetes who had to cut back their insulin shots. Keep in mind, all of this was accomplished with structural bodywork alone.

ASKING THE BODY FOR ANSWERS

As our reputation grew, the cases became tougher. I began seeing people with very severe problems that structural approaches alone didn't solve. When one gets to be a little too self-satisfied, God enters with greater challenges. I had learned how to ask the body to tell us what was wrong with it, using applied kinesiology, or muscle response testing.

Muscle testing is based on the premise that the body has an innate wisdom and can tell you what it needs. Through muscle testing, we found the body had holes in its energy field because of nutritional deficiencies and toxicities. We also found that emotional stresses were playing a major part in robbing us of our wellness. In fact, many people are held hostage by their emotions and circumstances, not knowing they have options to change their scripts.

In applied kinesiology, we deepened our understanding of structural, nutritional and emotional problems. Of course, as Dr. Sheldon Deal always said, each new discovery adds one more piece to the puzzle...and the more we learn, the more we realize we still have to learn. Because of this, we've spent our lives and practices continuing our education and improving our understanding of how to help people. However, while we were gaining new awareness of how to heal, modern medicine was heading down a very different path.

WHY MODERN MEDICINE FAILS

With the exception of the great successes in emergency trauma care in the medical profession, it's no secret that modern medicine is failing to meet the needs of people with serious health problems. After billions have been spent on cancer research, no cures have emerged. The more money we throw at it, the less we get. But we do get a self-perpetuating money-draining machine.

The reasons are well documented by the author of *The Cancer Industry*, Dr. Ralph Moss. Conflicts of interest are created when board members of pharmaceutical companies also sit on the committees overseeing drug approval, while also sitting on the boards that govern TV and other media sources of information. Rather than getting reliable information on the newest advances in health care, we get advertising disguised as news to market drugs and vaccines. Too much money is at stake for it to be otherwise.

Some feel even the FDA, fathered by Harvey Wiley to protect the consumer and patient, was overpowered from day one by massive commercial interests. Health protection for consumers of the food and drug industries was lost in favor of protecting the commercial interests of the drug and food companies.

ONLY "WELLNESS CARE" CAN PROTECT THE CONSUMER

Medicine cannot keep up with the crisis in degenerative health conditions of modern civilization. At the core of its failure is the simple fact that modern medicine provides disease care, not health care. It focuses on ever-smaller specialties and ever-smaller entities of disease and dysfunction. At best, you get symptomatic relief, but causes go unaddressed. Disease care is the fastest-growing failing business in America, to the tune of $1.3 trillion in 2002. Now it's over $2 trillion.

Over one-third of all patients surveyed by *The New England Journal of Medicine* have chosen alternative health care.

TOXIC AMERICA

While tranquilizers and antidepressants offer limited relief, the side effects have accumulated and added to our body's already overburdened systems. Emergency treatments of serious bacterial infections have enjoyed temporary success in ameliorating the conditions, but have also fostered new generations of drug-resistant strains of microbes that are more resistant to any treatment.

Many of our drug-resistant bugs are hatched in sewers. People dump their unused antibiotics in the toilet, unintentionally creating super-bugs.

Half of all antibiotics sold go into animal feed for our livestock – not to fight infection, but to increase weight gain for greater profitability and to prevent them from getting diseases. When we eat the meat, we're taking those antibiotics into our systems as well.

We are paying a price. All of this has helped create an overburdened body filled with toxic accumulations. This can cause a leaky gut, a toxic liver and/or an immune system to be over or underactive, each with its own set of listed symptoms and named diseases.

We now have a situation where almost everyone is subject to allergies as a result of an overburdened, toxic body. While we spend more and more on conventional health care, we get less and less. Costs have spiraled so much out of control that industry itself cannot afford to pay the bill.

Some mistakenly believe the answer is national or government-paid insurance known as "health care." Why can't we learn from countries that have almost totally bankrupted themselves trying that approach? We would still be getting "disease care" and not "health care." The system is flawed and will bankrupt whoever tries to pick up the tab.

A CURE FOR OUR HEALTH SYSTEM

Too much of the focus of conventional medicine has been on disease, and not enough attention has been given to wellness and health. Treatment of chronic disease conditions now amounts to 78-85% of our national health care bill in the U.S.

We spend little or nothing to find and treat the causes of disease, and little or nothing to find what prevents disease in the first place. And yet while all of this is taking place, more and more evidence accumulates showing the causes lie in our lifestyles: our polluted air, water, food, and our thoughts and actions. We, our cars and industries, have fouled our own nests with the thousands of chemical pollutants found in our processed foods, the depleted and poisoned soils we grow our foods in, the hormones, antibiotics and pesticides we subject our livestock to, the ocean of electromagnetic pollution we live in from our high-power electric wires, the electric appliances we depend on, the TVs and phones we use for communication, and the stresses from pollutants in our furniture and our workplaces.

The practitioners of holistic and wellness health care have resurrected the good principles that have been a part of our civilization for thousands of years, an ancient wisdom that believed in the natural harmony and balance of all things, a wisdom that knew the intelligence of the Creator was found naturally in the creation, as long as it wasn't interfered with.

Recognition of the life forces and innate intelligence of all living things was fundamental to traditional Chinese medicine, Indian Ayurvedic medicine, and to the founder of modern medicine, Hippocrates. It was also at the foundation of the philosophy of Daniel Palmer, the father of chiropractic.

Spirituality, mental balance, calmness, proper diet, healthy work and home environment, physical exercise and positive attitudes were all shared by the holistic health care of our past and by the *true* health care practitioners found in the wellness care of our present. What insurance companies have called health care has always been *disease* care.

In fact, they assign a disease code number you must list on the claim to get it paid. Then, we have to let them decide how much they might pay, or whether they're going to pay at all. Sometimes, the insurance companies decide you didn't need the care you may have already received, in which case, the insurance companies may further decide that doctors won't get paid for work they've already done. And for all that, we have to pay our insurance companies in advance.

Insurance companies by design are not in business to keep you well. They are in business to make a profit. It must be up to *YOU* to get and stay well! Our health and wellness are our responsibility. If we contract with a company to help us achieve that, then we had better be sure they cover wellness and not disease care.

Just look at the question patients ask when seeing a wellness practitioner – "Will you accept my insurance coverage?" This question misses the whole point. It's not that practitioners won't take insurance; it's that the insurance companies won't take the wellness practitioner. Not unless you force them. In the meantime you may have to pay cash. Remember, insurance companies don't want to pay any claim.

THE GOOD NEWS

Insurance companies will have to listen to consumers if you speak loud enough. And you, the consumer, can make your voice heard. If you always do what you've always done, you'll always get what you always gotten. If you want something different, read this book. The solution lies within to create health and wellness.

With our ancient traditions, we believe our minds and bodies know how to take care of themselves unless there is interference. The picture of wellness begins to emerge if we look at the whole person, evaluate if there is any interference with this whole person, and then put the pieces of the puzzle together.

We've identified *6 Interferences To Health* and *6 Steps To Wellness* in our health care. By implementing the *6 Steps To Wellness*, we can remove the *6 Interferences To Health*, thereby healing the body the way it was meant to be healed ... naturally.

6 Interferences To Health

1. Structural
2. Electromagnetic
3. Nutritional
4. Allergies
5. Emotional
6. Toxic Accumulations

6 Steps To Wellness

Step 1: Re-establish Structural Integrity:
      The Foundation of Health

Step 2: Rebalance Electromagnetics

Step 3: Rebalance Nutrition
    A. Reset Adrenals and the General Adaptive System
    B. Replenish Nutrition for Organ, Glands or System Weakness
    C. Reduce Infective Organisms in the Body
    D. Replace Enzymes and/or HCL to Aid Digestion, Assimilation and Elimination
    E Restore Proper Bowel Flora to Optimize Colon Function

Step 4: Reprogram the Body for any Allergies/ Sensitivities

Step 5: Re-evaluate Emotional Patterns and
          Remove Limiting Belief Systems
Step 6: Remove Heavy Metals or Other Toxins
          from the Body

• •

The essence of this book, and our practice, is simple. There are 6 causes of illness or avenues of interference that, when removed, the body can return to wellness...and the 6 Steps To Wellness contribute to the removal of these interferences.

We hope for miracles, and we see them many times. Do we always get them? No, unfortunately, we don't. Do we offer people false hope and empty promises? No, we simply offer the best, most complete health care available. This isn't just our occupation. It's our obsession. We feel it is our calling to help people achieve the health and wellness they deserve.

The book is intended for the general reader, but also contains terms and instruction aimed at holistic health practitioners. Don't let the occasional medical terms confuse you. Go with the flow.

We invite you to read this book with an open mind. As Bernie Segal, MD, said, "There is no such thing as an incurable disease, although there are incurable people."

In wellness care, we don't treat conditions that have people; we treat people who have conditions. We don't treat cancer ... we treat people with cancer. We don't treat MS or FM or CFS or carpal tunnel syndrome...we treat *people* with these conditions. We treat what and where the body tells us too. The conditions may very well be able to take care of themselves, provided we correct the *6 Interferences To Health* through the *6 Steps To Wellness*.

— John W. Brimhall, DC & Brett B. Brimhall, DC

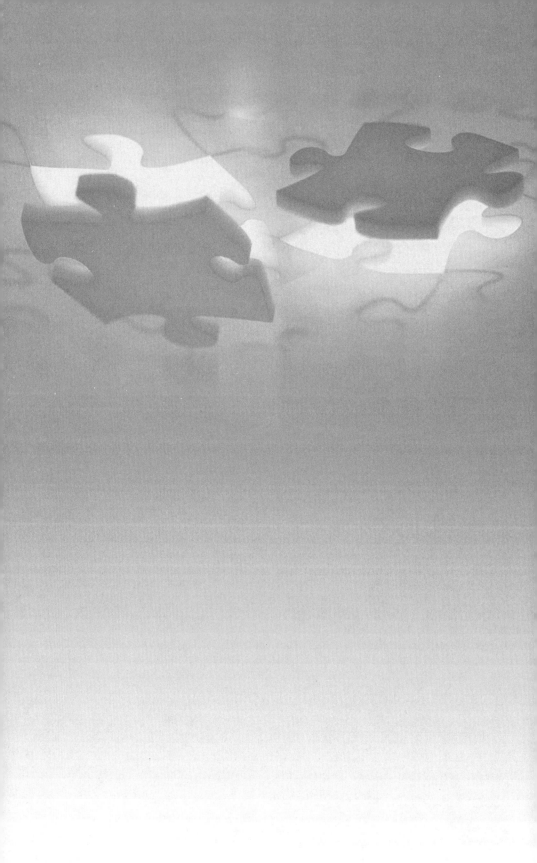

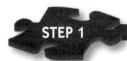

RE-ESTABLISH STRUCTURAL INTEGRITY: THE FOUNDATION OF HEALTH

BODY, HEAL THYSELF

Our body has an intelligence that knows how to take care of itself, provided it does not have interference from the six possible causes of disease: Structure, Electromagnetics, Nutrition, Emotions, Allergies or Toxic accumulation.

When nerves, lymph, cerebral spinal fluid, blood or acupuncture meridians are blocked by spinal misalignment or fixation, the life energy to all other systems, tissues and organs is interfered with. When blockages in the fascia, or connective tissue exist, the body stands in its own way, unable to give or receive accurate signals.

The heart and brain generate the greater part of the electrical energy of the whole body. In *Energy Medicine in Therapeutics and Human Performance*, Dr. James Oschman documents that every time the heart pulsates, it produces electrical energy to help create and balance the energy field that promotes health and wellness. All organs and systems must work unimpeded. When life energy is blocked through structural subluxation, fixation or scar tissue, you have malfunction. This may happen at the spinal column, extremities, craniosacral area, acupuncture meridians, at any organ, or scar tissue from any surgery, accident or emotional stress.

For example, a blockage may cause interference with blood circulation, and all the processes the body uses to eliminate its own wastes and toxins will be compromised.

In his work with applied kinesiology, Dr. George Goodheart has taught us that vertebral subluxations cause interruption of cerebral spinal fluid flow, interrupt nerve communication, impede lymph and blood circulation and cause interference in acupuncture meridians. Remove these interferences, find where the switches are turned off, turn them back on, and the body has the ability to heal itself. 80% of all conditions improve when the structure of the body is properly re-established.

Tools of the Trade

Many modern breakthrough tools now exist to rebalance the body easily, naturally, and safely, and help restore it to wellness — all without the discomfort of many styles of bodywork. Examples of these tools:

- The Erchonia® Adjustor (spinal)
- Percussor (cranial/fascial)
- 635 nm Low Level Laser
- 405 nm (violet) Low Level Laser

Re-establishing the structural integrity of the body is the foundation of health. We see more miracles with structural correction than any other form of treatment. We've also seen that to maintain these miracles, one must solve each of the 6 pieces of the interference puzzle.

If you correct the spine, fascia and/or craniosacral motion and still have nutritional deficiencies, allergies/sensitivities, toxic accumulations, unresolved emotions or electromagnetic pollution, then the structural problem returns. The real miracle comes when you and the wellness practitioner put all pieces of the puzzle together at the same time. Always remember, "Health is not a destination — it's a journey."

MISALIGNMENTS

Adjustment of the spine has been with us since Egyptian times. Daniel Palmer, a student of anatomy and physiology, founded the modern system and theory of chiropractic in 1895.

Can You Hear Me Now?

Daniel Palmer met a janitor who had been deaf for 17 years following an injury to his upper spine.

On examination, Palmer found a misaligned vertebra which corresponded to the area the janitor had injured 17 years before. By adjusting the vertebra and bringing it back into normal alignment, Palmer restored the janitor's hearing.

• •

WISDOM OF THE BODY

Palmer developed a philosophy that health was the normal state of the body when structure and function were in perfect equilibrium. He believed that all living things were endowed with "innate intelligence." Palmer theorized that this intelligence flows through the central nervous system and regulates all the organs, systems and vital functions of the body. It "knows" how to keep the body in health.

Palmer felt the purpose of the chiropractor was to remove nerve interference caused by spinal misalignments that blocked or restricted the intelligence of the body from carrying out its natural role of healthy regulation.

The task of the doctor was not to treat conditions, but to re-establish the structural integrity of the body. The chiropractor wasn't considered the healer. The doctor simply removes interference, permitting the body to heal itself naturally.

LIGHTS ON, LIGHTS OFF

Life force flows through the nerves to all cells and organs. If the system is interrupted, the body may communicate warnings as pain and other symptoms, indicating transmission from brain to body or body to brain has been interfered with. Let's oversimplify the process and look at it like a light switch. If the switch is on, the light works. If the switch is off, the light doesn't work. Turn any of these switches off, and you get a disorder in a corresponding system of the body. When the interference is removed, the body heals itself from within.

STRUCTURE RULES FUNCTION

In the early stages of chiropractic, some believed that misalignments of the spine were the only cause of disease. Today we understand there are many pieces of the puzzle that constitute wellness, which we have put together into 6 Steps.

Spinal, skeletal, muscular and connective-tissue structural misalignments are major components that can be adjusted to remove interference and allow the body to heal itself. When the structure is right, we see 80% of all conditions improve. Re-establishing structural integrity is still the foundation of health.

Today chiropractic is a champion of holistic and wellness health care and has become the world's second-largest health care field. Each year, over 15 million people choose chiropractic health care for natural, drug-free approaches to internal conditions, pain, backaches, injuries and trauma. Remember, we don't treat conditions that have people, we treat people who have conditions. And we see miracles happen every day by treating the whole person, not the disease.

• • • • • • • • • • • • • • • • • • • •

The Foundation of Health

Structure does rule function. Therefore, we must have balanced structure in all parts of the body. There are also three nervous systems that must be in balance:

1. The central nervous system, including brain and spinal cord
2. The peripheral nervous system, connecting the central nervous system to muscles and body tissues
3. The autonomic nervous system, which controls involuntary functions of organs, glands and digestion.

• • • • • • • • • • • • • • • • • • • •

THE SPINAL CONNECTION

All three of our nervous systems have connections to the spinal column, made up of 24 vertebrae that protect and surround the spinal chord. Between each of these vertebrae, pairs of nerves emit and extend to every part of the body's glands, organs, muscles and bones. The cranium and brain sit on top of the spine, while the hip bones attach to the bottom of the spine, connecting it to the lower extremities.

• •

Cervical (Neck) Vertebrae and Their Connections

1-C: Blood supply of the head, pituitary gland, scalp, bones of face, brain, middle ear and sympathetic nervous system

2-C: Eyes, auditory nerves, sinuses, mastoid bones, tongue, forehead

3-C: Cheeks, outer ear, face bones, teeth, trifacial nerve

4-C: Nose, lips, mouth, Eustachian tube

5-C: Vocal cords, neck glands, pharynx

6-C: Neck muscles, shoulders and tonsils

7-C: Thyroid, shoulders, elbows

Thoracic (Back) Vertebrae and Their Connections:

1-T: Arms and hands from the elbow down, wrists and fingers, esophagus and trachea

2-T: Heart and coronary arteries

3-T: Lungs, bronchial tubes, chest and breast

4-T: Gallbladder

5-T: Liver, solar plexus and blood

6-T: Stomach

7-T: Pancreas and duodenum

8-T: Spleen

9-T: Adrenal and supra-renal glands

10-T: Kidneys

11-T: Kidneys and ureters

12-T: Small intestines and lymph circulation

Lumbar (Lower Back) Vertebrae and Their Connections
- 1-L: Large intestine and inguinal rings
- 2-L: Appendix, abdomen and upper leg
- 3-L: Sex organs, uterus, bladder and knees
- 4-L: Prostate, lower back muscles and sciatic nerve
- 5-L: Lower legs, ankle and feet

Tailbone Connections
Tailbone: hipbones, buttocks, rectum and anus

· ● ● ● ● ●

THE HIP BONE'S CONNECTED TO THE BACK BONE
Each part of the spine can affect many parts of the body. Lower back pain can force a person to adjust by bending forward, placing pressure on the upper part of the back. This causes neck muscles to contract, which can lead to vision problems and headaches.

Dr. Oschman's research reports evidence of another nervous system referred to as the Continuum Pathway, which arrives from the connective tissue, thought by many to be a liquid crystalline, holographic structure.

This concept allows us to see the connective-tissue matrix as the largest organ of the body and the interconnection of all nervous systems: it's a structure that communicates at almost instantaneous, faster-than-nerve-conduction speeds to every part of the living matrix with laser-like, coherent communication.

This explains why we get what seem like miracle cures using the 635 nm (nanometer) Erchonia laser, which basically talks to the body's living matrix in its own language. We've also learned that pharmaceutical-grade, synergistic nutrition can communicate with the living matrix in similar ways.

● ● ● ● ● ● ● ● ● ● ● ● ● ● · · · · ·

ENTER THE MATRIX
In the forward to one of Dr. Oschman's books, *Energy Medicine in Therapeutics and Human Performance,* Dr. Karl Maret states that cells in

energy medicine are seen as fractals embedded in a holographic, energetic matrix where everything is interconnected and capable of influencing any other part of the matrix. He further states that information can be communicated through light, sound, color, vibration and quantum potentials.

"Ultimately," Maret wrote, "a picture of an electromagnetically unified matrix containing a self-organizing blueprint with innumerable feedback loops begins to emerge." We use all of this information to identify and eliminate any of the "6 Interferences" to allow you and your family to have the health and wellness you deserve.

. . . .

Now we see why many conditions improve with chiropractic adjustment, including bronchial asthma, sinus problems, high blood pressure, heart problems, GI disorders, respiratory conditions, impaired speech, angina caused by misalignment of cervical and thoracic vertebrae, and the common cold.

Misalignment of the lower back can cause many sexual problems that clear up when nerve interference is removed. This also helps explain why *6 Steps To Wellness* gives results when many other single treatments have failed. We're influencing the entire living matrix with –

- Nutrition
- Emotional release techniques
- Color
- Percussion of the fascia and scar tissue
- Sound, vibration
- 635 nm Low Level Laser
- 405 nm (violet) Low Level Laser
- Detoxification
- Energy balance

THE ERCHONIA ADJUSTOR

An elderly woman came to see us after undergoing an expensive operation for carpal tunnel syndrome that left her with all the same problems she suffered before the operation. With muscle response testing, we identified where the cause of the problem existed.

• •

The body holds all the wisdom it needs to heal itself.

• •

The woman couldn't hold her finger and thumb together in an O-ring. Her strength was severely diminished in her hands and wrists. In fact, her wrist extensors were very weak when tested as well. We found poor range of motion in both arms and shoulders. We found three neck vertebrae that were locked up or fixated. The switches were turned off. We did a very light adjustment with the Erchonia Adjustor instrument.

The Erchonia Adjustor, an instrument we co-invented, gives the body a light tapping motion that accomplishes what traditional chiropractic's thrusting adjustments accomplish. It's easier for the practitioner and usually causes no discomfort for the patient.

Immediately her pain was relieved. Her flexibility dramatically improved. Her strength returned to her hands and fingers. This was far more than the expensive operation had accomplished, and it only took a few moments.

• •

Right Body Structure

Dr. Goodheart has always taught that God will forgive you, but your nervous system will not. Structure rules function, and movement is life. The foundation of health has to be restored first, and that means making the structure of the body right.

• •

Complete healing of the woman's carpal tunnel syndrome took several more weeks, supported by the other five steps to wellness, including nutritional support and neutralizing the electromagnetic field disturbance that can be one of the causes of these kinds of injuries.

It's rare, indeed, to need surgery for carpal tunnel now that we have the Erchonia Adjustor, Percussor, cold laser and specific nutrition. Many times, the real cause of the problem is not in the wrist, but could be in the neck, elbow, scar tissue, acupuncture meridians, etc.

• •

The Real Cause of Carpal Tunnel Syndrome

Have you ever wondered why secretaries, who work with manual typewriters, seldom develop carpal tunnel syndrome, even though it takes more muscular effort than computer keyboards?

Computer keyboards take very light touches and require very little muscular effort, causing aches, pains and stiffness for everyone who uses them, frequently leading to carpal tunnel syndrome.

The stress on the body is caused by the electromagnetic field of the computer. (See Step 2: Rebalance Electromagnetics for a full explanation.) There are very simple, inexpensive devices that can protect you from these stresses and prevent many injuries and disorders as well as reverse them. With additional specific adjustments, cold laser and nutritional support, one can expect 90% of carpal tunnel and similar syndromes to improve or to become completely well.

• •

MIRACLES DO HAPPEN

Many body disturbances are resolved with spinal, extremity, visceral and scar tissue adjustment, including joint pains in hands, elbows, hips, shoulders, spine, and pain in other locations. Conditions such as fibromyalgia, arthritic problems, menstrual difficulties, bursitis, as well as a wide range of emotional disorders from mild depression to schizophrenia, respond because structural correction is one of the *6 Steps To Wellness* that corrects the cause of the disease but doesn't chase any of the symptoms of the condition. We see miracles happen every day.

• • • • • • • • • • • • • • • • • • •

A Letter About Lower Back Pain

Dear T. Grade, MD

I want to thank you for referring me to Dr. Brimhall last fall. I haven't had to use the walker since I started to go to him and was even able to start work in February. I didn't think I'd ever be able to stay right-end-up long enough to keep a job again. You were right. He was able to find out what was causing the problem and has come a long way toward fixing it. It amazes me that he was able to find it when no one else could. The pain in the lower back and hips was caused by the L5 being twisted. What a shock it was to have the pain go away for the first time in nearly two years. Dr. Grade, I finally have my life back.

— Marianne

• • • • • • • • • • • • • • • • • • •

Combined with nutritional therapy, dietary changes and exercise, chiropractic has improved and sometimes helped reverse osteoarthritis. Population studies in Australia considered chiropractic more helpful in alleviating problems with post-polio syndrome than any other treatment. Britain's Medical Research Council found chiropractic more helpful than hospital outpatient care for lower back pain.

In costs of treatment, the Worker's Compensation Fund found that the fund spent 10 times more for medical care than it did for chiropractic to treat back pain, generally. In addition, the time spent for medical care requires longer treatment periods.

Work habits, repetitive motions, posture, the ergonomics of the work place, the electromagnetic fields of the workplace, diet, family history, exercise or sedentary habits, environmental pollutants, air quality, water intake, caffeine, smoking and alcohol intake are all taken into consideration in determining the steps you need to take to restore or maintain health.

All of the following play important roles in our holistic health care's *6 Steps To Wellness:*

- Spinal and craniosacral treatment
- Massage and rehabilitation exercises
- Applied kinesiology
- Acupuncture and meridian therapy
- Cold laser therapy
- Percussion myofascial release
- Therapeutic detox baths
- Infrared sauna
- Pure water
- Color therapy
- Sound therapy
- Emotional reprogramming
- Nutritional support

• • • • • • • • • • • • • • • • • • • •

A Grateful Client

Dear Dr. Brimhall,

So often people make time to complain, but never make time to give thanks. Since I have not had a chance to meet you in person, I just wanted to take a moment and express my appreciation to you and your entire staff. My father is a chiropractor and was very concerned when I was in my automobile accident. He met you and was relieved when he found out that your office was located so close to me. Your chiropractic assistants have been great. I had never received massage therapy before. Cindy often had to work in deep muscle tissue in my neck, which wasn't very fun, but the mobility in my neck would double after each treatment, and it helped me to sleep so much better. There was a major release in my back. I would say 60% of the pain and stiffness was gone. For the headaches Dr. Kirkman thoroughly worked over my cranium and my neck, and I had 90% relief! I really appreciate your efforts to offer such advanced health care. You truly have established a one-of-a-kind clinic, and I feel privileged to have experienced it.

— Kristy

ERCHONIA COLD LASER

The cold laser can do almost everything acupuncture needles can do for pain, without you feeling a thing.

The Erchonia cold laser emits a ruby-red light that can correct misalignments in the spine so gently that you feel nothing. The same gentle approach can release stress patterns in the fascia (fibrous tissue surrounding your organs, muscles and other soft structures) quickly and painlessly.

The laser, when used above your skin on an area of injury, pain or trauma, rapidly reduces pain and swelling and accelerates healing at dramatic rates that were only dreamed of in the past.

German physicist and biophysicist, Fritz Albert Popp, was the first to identify the frequency of the biophoton radiation, which radiates from the human body at 635 nanometers (nm). This biophoton radiation belt extends about an inch and a half around the average person, extending further around the heart and head, much as

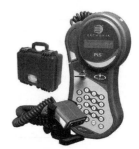

Erchonia Cold Laser
www.brimhall.com

50

religious paintings show halos (auras) around the heads of spiritual people.

The Erchonia diode laser emits the same wavelength of frequency as the healthy human body, 635 nm. This amazing tool is called the cold laser, soft laser, low-power laser or the low-level laser.

• • • • • • • • • • • • • • • • • • •

Lasers

The term LASER is an acronym for Light Amplification by Stimulated Emissions of Radiation. Lasers emit coherent, focused light that travels in a narrow beam in one direction. High-power or "hot" lasers have larger, higher energy waves with catabolic effects that can deliberately destroy tissue in cauterizing and surgical applications. Low-power, "soft," "cool," or "cold" lasers have lower power, smaller waves with anabolic effects that promote rapid reduction of pain, accelerate healing time, and accelerate growth and repair.

· · · · · · · · · · · · · · · · · · · •

Cold lasers aren't capable of producing thermal damage in tissue. Cold lasers have balancing effects rather than destructive ones. They're totally safe for both doctor and patient without negative side effects.

My first experience with laser treatment in the 1970s proved to me that the cold laser could do everything the needle in acupuncture could do, far better than acupressure or magnets, which also restore electromagnetic fields.

We also discovered that the laser could be used on acupuncture meridians and points as well as many spinal misalignments with dramatic therapeutic effects. Combined with synergies among nutritional and other treatment modalities, we have achieved success rates ranging from 70-90%.

LCDS AND LIVING ORGANISMS

Liquid crystalline structures are ideal for LCD computer display screens because they respond readily to changes in electric and biomagnetic fields. Liquid crystals are tunable, responsive systems; even high-definition TV screens are made with LCD technology.

Quantum physics states that all of the major constituents of living organisms may also be liquid crystalline in nature. The collagen alignments in connective tissue (which have a liquid crystalline mix of collagen and bound water) are thought to be tied closely and interconnect with the acupuncture systems of meridians and points. These acupuncture meridians and points are said to be electromagnetic transmission lines of communication on which the health and well-being of the body depend, much like the nerves in the central nervous system communicate with and feed the body's organs and systems.

Mae-Wan Ho, in her book "The Rainbow and The Worm," has suggested that only weak electromagnetic fields optimally stimulate the body's healing and regeneration actions, which are triggered by this liquid crystalline matrix of connective tissue. Photons from the Erchonia cold laser communicate with the cells on the same 635 nm wavelength the cells themselves use.

LIQUID CRYSTALLINE MATRIX AND COLD LASER

Power lines, computers, hair dryers, cell phones, etc., disturb our energy fields and are thought to be a major cause of our modern-day illnesses. The cold laser restores the cells' optimum weak electromagnetic field. Cold laser may be the optimum low-frequency tool for best results in this triggering mechanism, surpassing mechanical, heat and other means.

Like an LCD, this crystalline matrix communicates with the whole body, has a memory, and responds to new information. As J.B. Glazewski noted in *Low-energy laser therapy as quantum medicine, Laser Therapy*, local application of laser irradiation can be observed in anatomically distant parts and organs. The beneficial effects at the irradiated site extend elsewhere in the body.

HEALING ALLERGIES WITH COLD LASER

For allergies, we found the laser can duplicate or improve the beneficial effects reported in some cultures where people ritually hold their food, or hold their hands above the food they're going to eat. They're tuning the food to the 635 nm frequency of the human body. In a similar way, we ask people to hold the food (or vial containing the substance) they were allergic to – for example, wheat – then cold laser the wheat in the hand to "rewrite the script" in the body's memory so the person is no longer sensitive to the food or allergen.

The combination of body-allergen and laser irradiation neutralizes the allergenic effect on the patient. We've oversimplified this procedure here and will do it more justice under the allergy section. The technique is called A/SERT (Allergy/Sensitivity Elimination and Reprogramming Technique).

Mae-Wan Ho has a fine explanation. The frequency of each object oscillates with every other object in any given place. One object absorbs the oscillating frequency of the other until they're coupled in the same frequency. Note these examples from nature:

- Crickets chirping in unison
- Fireflies flashing together in perfect time
- The pacemaker cells of the heart
- The insulin-secreting cells of the pancreas

All are synchronized electrical activities.

COLD LASER DIAGNOSIS AND TREATMENT

The cold laser can be used in both diagnosis and treatment. Brief use of the Erchonia 635 nm laser over the site of an injury or disorder will strengthen reflexes and muscles, increase range of motion and reduce pain. Longer irradiation of the same site helps restore healthy function.

Different frequencies are suspected to trigger the release of heavy metals. The electromagnetic signatures of metals were researched and recorded by Dr. Max Collins. When the Erchonia cold laser is adjusted to mimic these frequencies, the body releases the metals, sometimes so rapidly you can smell them on your breath or taste a metallic taste. The same is true of infectious organisms. Their frequencies are also known, and the right laser frequency may help eliminate a virus, bacteria or parasite from the body.

The cold laser provides you with a patient-friendly tool that can accomplish many therapeutic ends, diminish pain, increase circulation of blood and lymph, and accelerate the growth and repair mechanisms of the human body.

Cold laser applications may help explain why synergistic effects are far greater than any single-treatment mode when tissues are lasered and nutritional therapies are combined.

• •

Cold Laser Applications

The cold laser is a perfect conjunctive tool for:

- Chiropractors
- Medical Doctors
- Acupuncturists
- Physical Therapists

Clinical applications of the cold laser have included:

- Acute and chronic pain reduction from many causes
- Inflammation reduction
- Enhanced tissue healing
- Cell regeneration
- Replacement of the needle in acupuncture

The results have shown very rapid pain reduction, accelerating recovery times by 25-40%, far exceeding conventional methods.

• •

PAIN THERAPY

We see miracles every day when cold laser irradiation is applied to sites of pain and related accupoints. The treatments have produced positive results for:

- Tension headaches
- TMJ
- Neck and shoulder aches
- Sprains
- Frozen shoulder
- Chest pains such as Tietze's syndrome
- Tennis elbow
- Osteoarthritis pain in hands and hips
- Sciatic pain
- Achilles tendonitis
- Knee joint pain
- Ankle sprains
- Fasciitis plantaris

The Case of Dr. J.M.

Dr. J.M. had suffered with 25 years of neck pain from a frozen neck. Traditional chiropractic adjustments once a week had helped him cope with the pain, but it remained unresolved and his neck would still go out on him when he moved it slightly the wrong way. In just minutes of lasering his neck muscles to his shoulder muscles – 60 seconds on the left, another 60 on the right – the muscles relaxed and released. He reported that the sensation of stiff heaviness felt "light" and weightless immediately. A healthy range of motion was restored, and he was pain-free.

The Case of Dr. J.E.

Dr. J.E. suffered chronic lower-back pain for at least 7-10 years and had suffered a stiff back and stiff legs for "a lifetime." In high school, his participation in sports was severely restricted by stiffness. On examination, he was unable to bend over further than his hands reaching the level of his knees. After cold laser treatment, he bent over to touch the floor. It was the first time he remembered ever having that much flexibility.

The Case of Dr. R.G.

Dr. R.G. had lost his sense of smell for 20 years. After one laser treatment to release the blocks in corresponding nerves, his sense of smell returned.

CLINICAL STUDIES

Cold laser irradiation has shown significant improvement in many fibromyalgia (FM) patients in the clinical and quality-of-life indicators:

- Alleviation of pain
- Reduction of number of tender points
- Improvements in skin-fold tenderness
- Morning stiffness
- Sleep disturbance
- Muscular spasm
- Fatigue
- Depression

We've seen miraculous improvements in everything involving pain from FM to Multiple Sclerosis. The as-yet undiscovered uses may be endless.

ANOTHER TREATMENT FOR CARPAL TUNNEL SYNDROME

We spoke earlier of a carpal tunnel syndrome patient responding to adjusting with the Erchonia Adjustor. Cold laser also offers a very effective treatment.

Carpal tunnel syndrome (CTS) and repetitive stress injury (RSI) have become common conditions in office workers using desktop computers, meat cutters, auto assemblers, musicians playing stringed instruments, and other groups where mechanically repetitive motions are performed throughout the workday. Those who are affected frequently experience pain, numbness, tingling in hands and wrists as well as in thumb, index and middle fingers. Those diagnosed with CTS or RSI also show neuromuscular problems in the head, neck and upper back upon examination.

Symptoms lasting from months to years in a group of 35 patients diagnosed with CTS or RSI had been treated by various medical and other health care modalities without pain relief. All patients had varying degrees of abnormal posture with forward, rounded shoulders, and head and neck stooped forward. All patients showed tenderness when touched in the lower and upper spine. Each tender site in the spine (but not the wrists or hands) was treated for two to five minutes with a cold laser touching the skin. Each patient was followed for about three months, averaging 10 treatments per patient. Instruction in posture and proper ergonomics was also given, and in some instances, harnesses or collars were employed.

Pain, numbness and tingling in hands and wrists subsided or disappeared in all patients, and none of the patients reported adverse effects or worsening in symptoms. Some patients experienced immediate relief, less pain and tingling in arms, hands and fingers, less tenderness in lower and upper spine, and greater muscle relaxation. Among the 35 treated, one was pain-free after three treatments; others saw symptoms clear up in less than three months.

In most of these cases diagnosed as CTS or RSI, the patients also remembered long-ago sports injuries, automobile accident injuries or injuries from falls. It was believed that prolonged straining of these old injuries by improper posture and ergonomics aggravated and perpetuated old microscopic or macroscopic tears in soft tissues, resulting in painful accumulation of chemicals such as histamine, kinins and other substances. The cold laser helps alleviate and drain these irritating chemicals through lymphatic channels.

In a 100-patient blind study, the Erchonia diode cold laser of ruby red, near-infrared light was tested on chronic neck and shoulder pain associated with osteoarthritis, muscle spasms or spinal sprain conditions. The cold laser was used for durations of 30-90 seconds, while the control group received placebo treatments with no irradiation from a "fake" laser. The results showed that 65% of the cold laser-treated group showed 30% improvement in pain, while only 11.6% of the placebo group improved to this degree.

In a clinical trial of another 100 subjects, the majority of the test group showed significant reduction in pain levels immediately following a single treatment. This pain reduction was stable or improved further after 24 hours. The test group receiving a single laser treatment also significantly improved in all ranges of motion, while the placebo group didn't show significant improvement.

COLD LASER IN SPORTS MEDICINE

Cold laser irradiation of sports injuries has resulted in rapid recoveries, profoundly benefiting the individuals' personal lives and athletic careers. In treatment of 57 athletic injuries including cuts, scrapes, strains and sprains, overuse conditions and stress reactions, 54 of the 57 showed dramatically positive reductions of pain levels and improvement in functional tests.

After six days of cold laser treatment, one soccer player was pain-free and completed the season without recurrence. A defensive lineman in football with chronic unresolved ankle sprain and infection began to heal, and the wound began to close after two laser treatments. After four treatments, the wound had healed. The athlete returned to competition 10 days earlier than the team physician had anticipated. Similar accelerated rates of wound healing have been noted in burn cases.

After one treatment of cold laser irradiation to trigger points and acupuncture points, another athlete reported a 50% reduction in pain. Two additional treatments on two consecutive days resulted in the patient becoming pain-free, with normal range of motion and normal strength.

These kinds of rapid improvements in pain management with cold laser stimulation have been attributed to stimulation of the mitochondria (the energy-producing part of a cell), leading to enhanced protein formation and energy. Also linked to cold laser stimulation are photochemical changes which reduce sensitivity of nerve endings and changes in biochemicals that have anti-inflammatory effects. These changes were accompanied by 30-50% improvement of collagen formation in wound healing.

COLD LASER APPLICATIONS

In dentistry, the cold laser has reduced dentin hypersensitivity to different irritating agents by as much as 60%. In conditions that involve spasm keeping the jaw tightly closed, beneficial results have been achieved. Positive postsurgical analgesic effects have been demonstrated that include problem-free post-operative periods and accelerated healing of operation wounds.

COLD LASERS AS PAIN RELIEVERS

Pain-killing effects are supported by laser-stimulated, enhanced circulation of blood and accelerated outflow of lymph from the region involved. Improved blood and lymph circulation also stimulate the body's ability to heal itself.

Laser irradiation improves temporary communication of pain signals across nerves. This is accompanied by laser-enhanced production of the body's own pain-killing opiates, the enkephalins. Together, these two biochemical actions are the equivalent of non-narcotic analgesia.

Pain sensors in most tissues (including skin, muscle, joint and mucosal membranes) are gateways for pain perception. Pain sensors at irritated sites are directly desensitized by laser irradiation. Lasers stimulate the release of the body's own opiates, alpha and beta endorphins, which bind to pain receptors at the site of irritation. Following local irradiation, pain chemical byproducts are increasingly eliminated in the urine. Transfer of pain information from the irritated site to the gray matter of the spine is also decelerated by laser irradiation. Transfer of information by peripheral nerves reduces irritability. On average, pain relief between 70-85% with the use of the laser alone has been demonstrated in about 80% of patients studied.

Laser light stimulates enhanced cellular energy, tissue oxygenation and nutrition, all of which accelerate wound healing.

COLD LASER ON NERVOUS SYSTEM INJURIES

Approximately 250,000 people in the United States today live with spinal cord injuries. These individuals experience different degrees of paralysis, sensory impairment, bowel, bladder and sexual dysfunctions that are believed to be irreversible. The majority of these people have lived with permanent disability and handicap, costing the U.S. $380 million a year, not to mention costs in lost careers and lost quality of life.

Dr. Semion Rochkind first studied crush injury of sciatic nerves in rat models in 1962. Lasering at the site of the injured nerve at 635 nm promoted the action potential to 70% of the normal, healthy pre-crush value. This frequency was found to have better penetration ability through the skin to reach injured nerves. This may be a preventative effect with human medical implications. A single laser treatment maintains the injured nerve at a high potential on the first day of injury. This is also true of laser irradiation of corresponding spinal cord segments, which are distant from the site of injury.

At the end of 360 days, a follow-up examination revealed the cold lasered group had much more functional feet, were devoid of ulcers and were well on their way to recovery. Histological studies of both the spinal cord and sciatic nerve showed no scar tissue formation in the spinal cord for the laser-treated group. The most important effect was prevention of the usual pathological changes seen in motor nerves. On Day 14 after the crush injury, the corresponding area in the spinal cord showed only minimal degenerative changes in 20% of the neurons, decreasing to 10% by Day 90.

Laser treatment of the injured nerve itself benefited the degenerative changes in the corresponding sections of the spinal cord, suggesting enhanced functioning of nerves and better physical nerve sheath formation, which led to faster regeneration of the distal nerve itself. Laser treatment of the spinal cord alone also improved the recovery of the injured nerve, enhancing the compound action potential of the nerve.

Laser irradiation was shown to stimulate the nerve-rebuilding substances and enhance production of other biochemicals. Both processes may have been responsible for facilitating the regeneration of the injured nerve and spinal cord.

STUDIES OF SPINAL CORD INJURIES

Dr. Rochkind applied his methods in clinical practice with seven human patients afflicted with tethered spinal cord, progressive motor or sensory losses in the legs, abnormal curvature of the spine, leg deformities and urinary tract dysfunction. Normally, the potential for reversal of these conditions is poor.

The tethered spinal cord and compressed nerve roots were surgically released, and laser treatment was given during the operation. The treatment increased the amplitude of evoked nerve responses from 15% to 52%.

The seven patients were followed for six months after treatment. During this time, their neurological status, gait disturbances and weakness in the lower extremities all improved. The degree of motor improvement was directly related to the length of time the symptoms of movement losses had existed prior to treatment. Two of the four scoliosis patients improved. Two of the three claw-foot cases improved. Five of the six cases with urinary incontinence and two with anal sphincter dysfunction showed progressive improvement. The attitude that damage is irreversible in old spinal cord injuries in humans must be reconsidered in light of the Rochkind et al studies through 2002. These gains with cold lasering are truly remarkable. Eight of his patients were treated six to eighteen months after injury. Two of the eight had paralysis affecting all four limbs, resulting from a fall and a gunshot wound. Two had paralyzed legs from Caisson Disease and an aviation accident. One had paralyzed legs and other motor weakness resulting from a road accident. Three had severe motor weakness from accidents and falls. Five of eight had sphincter paralysis.

Lasering from above the skin 4-6 inches with 635 nm wavelength significantly improved spinal cord conductivity in five of six spinal cord injuries and three with severe motor weakness. Two patients with bladder dysfunction and impaired sensation improved following laser treatment and regained voluntary ability to urinate and bladder control. All laser-treated patients had some degree of voluntary muscle improvement, the degree of which was directly related to the period of time the losses existed prior to treatment.

Patients were followed for four months, during which time five patients with urinary sphincter paralysis progressively improved. Two patients with severe muscle weakness returned to their former occupations.

CLINICAL STUDIES: LIPOSUCTION

Dr. Rodrigo Neira pioneered the use of the cold laser in liposuction surgery in 2000. After six minutes of above-the-skin exposure of 635 nm cold laser to fatty tissue treated with anesthesia, Neira et al found that almost 100% of the target fat had been liquefied, facilitating liposuction and making for an easier extraction, with less surgical trauma and better clinical results.

MRI images showed that after four minutes of laser irradiation, 80% of targeted fatty cells, which initially looked like clusters of grapes, had emulsified, causing fat to escape from inside the cell. After six minutes of exposure, the percentage of liquefaction increased to almost 100%. In later microscopic studies, the fatty cell was shown to develop a transitory pore, which allowed the fat to escape, facilitating reduced risk and improved quality of life for the patient.

The effects of the laser were localized, facilitating fat extraction and preserving the surrounding structure and capillaries. No adverse toxic events were observed during the procedure or afterward. The cold laser produces less surgical trauma for the patient. Bruises and swellings filled with blood clots were reduced, enhancing patient recovery.

In a study of 40 liposuction procedures, patients were used as their own controls. On one side of the body, the patient received just liposuction. On the other side, liposuction and cold laser irradiation were combined. Two weeks after surgery, the benefits of cold laser irradiation became noticeable. Sites of laser-treated surgery had less swelling, less abnormal hardening of tissues and less discomfort.

Used following surgery, the cold laser led to improved wound healing, rapid reduction in pain and improvement in the inflammatory process. Patients reported that they healed faster, had less drainage and experienced more comfort when the laser was used. Other observations noted smoother, softer skin, decreased bruising and less dimpling.

During treatment, the cold laser was held 4-6 inches from the skin. The patient felt nothing. When treatments were combined during and after the operation, patients fared even better than with one treatment alone. Cold lasering resulted in beneficial increased circulation and enhanced wound healing.

FACELIFTS AND PLASTIC SURGERY

Facelift patients also showed reduced scarring and accelerated healing time with postoperative irradiation with the cold laser.

Dr. Richard Amy, who pioneered the 100-person studies that resulted in FDA approval of the Erchonia cold laser, saw a female patient who had undergone complicated face reconstruction surgery. She came for cold laser therapy because the surgery had gone wrong.

Her face resembled something out of a horror story. Her skin was red, swollen, infected and dying. After treatment with the cold laser three times a day, five times a week, over a period of six weeks, the woman's face totally healed, and she had the new-looking, healthy skin she wanted in the first place.

CLINICAL STUDIES: OTHER SKIN INJURIES

The healing of diabetic ulcers, venous ulcers and skin injuries were studied in five patients who exhibited slow rates of wound closure. All patients had undergone months to years of conventional wound management with little or no improvement. Patients were given instruction on using laser treatment at home for 30 minutes each day on the site of the wound and to return to a medical center seven days later.

In the case of the venous ulcer that had not healed since 1958, the wound measured 8.29 square cm on April 2, 1997, before laser treatment. In three months, the ulcer shrank to 1.21 square cm. It resolved on October 29, 1997.

SUMMARY OF COLD LASER BENEFITS

We believe that cold laser treatment holds great promise for:
- Rapid pain relief
- Increased circulation

- Relaxation of stressed areas
- Release of toxins
- Enhanced healing of injuries to the spine, nerves, muscle, skin and tendons, even in circumstances of poor circulation

Skin conditions can heal in as little as 28 to 35 days. Wounds can heal in four weeks. Sprains and strains can heal in six weeks. Ligament and cartilage damage may take as long as six months. In all cases, the length of time it takes to heal is reduced by 25-40% in the studies we have seen and in our clinical experience.

Pain relief, restoration of range of motion, and the return of strength are nearly instantaneous. Structure rules function, and restored motion is life. The laser helps accomplish our goals for structural correction.

PERCUSSION

Three basic bodily rhythms have been identified:
- The cardiac rhythm of the heartbeat
- The respiratory rhythm of breathing
- The craniosacral rhythm that results from the increase and decrease in the volume of cerebrospinal fluid within and around the craniosacral system

A BRIEF HISTORY OF CRANIOSACRAL THERAPY

Craniosacral therapy originally monitored craniosacral rhythm, a subtle, wavelike motion (which ranges from 6 to 10 oscillating cycles per minute and is for the most part unaffected by heartbeat and breathing), to determine any restriction or dysfunction in the craniosacral system.

Doctors were taught to feel with their hands for the wavelike motions of this system for its unified movement. With an extremely sensitive touch, the physician was able to diagnose the movement of the system by locating critical sites of restriction in the cranium. William G. Sutherland, DO, popularized this sutural technique in the early twentieth century. The technique involves manipulating the sutures of the skull to ease pressure, increasing the mobility of cranial bones. By removing stress between the bones, the sutural technique normalizes the relationship of bones to each other, helping restore the craniosacral system to healthy balance.

In the 1920s, Major B. DeJarnette, DC, developed a technique that combined sutural, meningeal and reflex approaches after his work with Dr. William Sutherland, which became known as Sacro-Occipital Technique™ and craniopathy. DeJarnette recorded that many conditions improved with this technique, including anxiety, inflammation, asthma, cataracts, diabetes, impotence and constipation, when associated with restrictions.

In the 1970s, John Upledger, DO, pioneered the meningeal technique, which has become known as Craniosacral Therapy™. This technique focuses on finding tension and restriction in the connective tissue known as the fascia that lines the skull and the spinal canal. The therapist prompts a release by gently applying pressure with the hand and elongating the membranes.

DEVELOPMENT OF PERCUSSION TECHNIQUE

Unheralded by most medical writers, Robert Fulford, DO, had developed his own individual system of craniosacral therapy in the 1940s. Fulford's many years of clinical experience had convinced him that the "fascia was difficult to free by the hand alone." He believed he needed a motor to fully release some restrictions. Dr. Fulford first introduced a simple percussion instrument, Fordom's lapidary hammer, to Craniosacral Therapy in order to enhance craniosacral rhythms and free up breathing patterns.

This percussion technique focused on finding an area of restriction in the craniosacral system and tapping the area gently with the percussion hammer while monitoring the opposite side of the restricted area with the therapist's free hand. The monitoring hand works to restrict the movement of the body as it tries to unwind the distorted fascia back to a normal condition. The combination of percussive movement and monitoring hand restriction results in a deep energy release of tension that has long-lasting consequences.

Andrew Weil, MD, with whom we have lectured on the same platform several times, has praised Dr. Fulford as the, "healing magician of our time," a doctor who could successfully, "treat problems other doctors could not solve."

I was fortunate enough to be able to take two seminars from Dr. Fulford in 1991 and 1992, the only two seminars that he allowed chiropractors to attend. Dr. Fulford said trauma of any kind was stored in the fascia and created an energy sink that caused aberrant information throughout the body and led to illness. We can see, in light of new information now available about the living matrix, that Dr. Fulford was an unsung genius. Dr. Weil saw this genius and wrote about him in several of his books.

I presented my first paper on craniosacral therapy to the International College of Applied Kinesiology (ICAK) in 1993, merging the use of the percussion instrument with new and earlier work on the whole body. It's a great instrument and technique for all bodywork, from myofascial and visceral release to the cranial bones, spine, extremities and other parts of the system. It helps the body-worker remove distortions wherever they exist in the organism.

This new percussion work extends the field of manual medicine past the craniosacral system to visceral corrections, scar tissue problems, the spine, extremities and beyond. In fact, without taking into consideration the fascia and this holographic energetic matrix that we now know about, how could one really practice wellness evaluation or treatment?

We, along with our team of Certified Teachers, have further developed the Erchonia VP-3™ Percussion Instrument™ and techniques, which have become invaluable tools, used by hundreds of doctors and wellness practitioners. These techniques and other certified instruction is taught at approximately forty Nutri-West/ Brimhall Wellness Seminars each year.

Percussor
www.brimhall.com

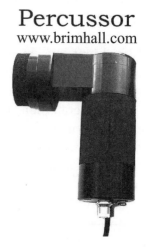

A Certified Wellness Practitioner in your area can be found by calling Brimhall Wellness Seminars at 866-338-4883.

Percussion and The Case of Dr. Kerra F.

In August of 1991, I was rear-ended by a car traveling 60 mph. I sustained multiple injuries including TMJ and a closed head injury. I lost my husband several months after the accident due to a fall from seizures (complications of his head injury). I had two TMJ surgeries, March 1992 and April 1994. I had returned to practice about a dozen times, always getting worse. I had given up on ever practicing again. In 1996, I was trying to sell my practice and was on full disability. I had several daily headaches with TMJ, a lower-back disc problem and major depression. Upon going to the CCA Convention (just to get my hours), my life changed when God led me to Dr. Brimhall. In front of a room full of chiropractors, Dr. Brimhall increased my range of motion of my TMJ by an inch. He made good on his promise. I returned to work in January 1997 for the first time in five years. I went back to work adding the percussor and nutritional supplements. I now spend 10 to 15 minutes per patient following Dr. Brimhall's protocol. My practice doubled within three months and we had 26 new patients in the month of August. Dr. Brimhall not only changed my health, but also helped my practice, therefore helping my patients.

— Dr. Kerra F.

PERCUSSION DISCUSSION

I took my first course from Dr. Fulford in 1991 and have not put down the percussor since. We have further developed many new uses for the new and improved percussion hammer.

Percussion is used for myriad conditions, including:

- Cranial suture fixations and misalignments
- Visceral manipulation

- Scar tissue adhesions and release
- Temporomandibular joint (TMJ) problems
- Spinal and pelvic misalignments and fixations
- Shoulder, elbow, wrist and hand problems
- Hip, knee, ankle and foot problems
- Acute and chronic sinus problems
- Lymphatic drainage congestion
- Craniosacral respiratory balancing
- Organ misplacement and fascial contractures
- Diaphragmatic spasm and hiatal hernia
- Release for emotionally related abdominal contractions.

Several generations of percussion instruments have progressed from the lapidary hammer to the Erchonia unit we now use, called the Brimhall Variable Percussor (VP-3).

The VP-3 Percussor's smooth, powerful action allows the therapist to work with the fascia of the body at a very deep, penetrating level that has long-lasting dimensions. We've found that fascial restrictions underlie many persistent misalignments of the spine, fixations, chronic pain syndromes and scar tissue. The penetrating force of this percussive action allows you to free both superficial connective tissue and the deep fascia.

There may be unlimited uses for the chiropractor, osteopath, Rolfer, therapist and related bodyworkers, as well as unlimited benefits for the patient. For instance, these percussion techniques can be used to:

- Align the spine
- Correct a TMJ
- Correct a spastic or incompetent ileocecal valve at the junction of the small and large intestine
- Release a spastic bowel
- Adjust the hips
- Adjust the lower extremities
- Adjust the knee joint
- Realign the connective tissue in the arch of the foot

Dr. Fulford's technique adjusted restrictions within the patient's body using a very light contact with the hammer at the restriction point and a more firm contact with the monitoring hand. For the most part, the monitoring hand is opposite the contact point and the driving line of the hammer. The body part being percussed then tries to unwind and stretch. The idea behind percussive connective tissue release involves restricting the unwinding and stretching action with the monitoring hand until a deep fascial-energy release is felt.

THE BODY ELECTRIC

Your bones and fascia have properties that let them carry electrical current. Fascial connective tissue is in constant communication with the entire nervous system.

Dr. Fulford believed the Craniosacral Fluid (CSF) was the highest force in man. It's formed in the brain and pumped by the rhythmic contraction of a part of the fascia called the dura mater – the sheath of connective tissue surrounding the brain and spine. The craniosacral system contracts 6-10 times per minute, and its cerebrospinal waves have far-reaching effects on sensory, motor and overall neurological functions. This system exists in all animals possessing a brain and spinal cord, forming in the womb and continuing to function until death.

Respiration has a bodily rhythm set to breathing patterns, just as the cardiovascular system is set to the rhythm of the heartbeat. They're independent of the CSF, yet related to and influenced by each other.

The cardiovascular system is very electric and uses blood vessels as signal transmitters. The heart acts not only as a mechanical pump, but also as a generator of electricity or charged ions throughout the whole body.

The fascial connective tissue around the heart is called the pericardium. Some researchers have referred to the pericardium as the body's main bank of stored electrical energy. Energy is also stored in the dura mater and other fascial connective tissue in lesser degrees.

When there's obstruction or resistance to this electrical flow of energy, the equilibrium that maintains all systems of the body becomes unbalanced, and malfunction may ensue.

The VP-3 percussion instrument has a strong enough motor for the mechanical force of its smooth vibrations to stimulate the release of the fascial connective tissue fully, through both biomechanical and bioelectric unwinding. This kind of release allows the fluids and electrical properties of tissues and organs to flow normally again, creating motion and life, restoring healthy equilibrium.

Dr. Fulford believed many of these obstructions originated as far back as early life in the womb or trauma from birth. His insights had come from careful observation of autopsies of infants and children, where he noticed severe adhesions and restrictions in cranial fascial connective tissue and the sheath of connective tissue surrounding the spine even at this early age.

PHYSICAL TRAUMA AND "ENERGY SINK"

The electrical forces passing through the patient determine the patterns of collagen-based fascial fibers. Any trauma, including emotional trauma, is an electrically charged event which can influence our bodily make-up.

According to Wolff's Law, our tissues grow and regenerate according to the demands placed upon them. Based on this law, traumas are recorded events in the tissues of the body. These recorded traumas can cause what's called an "energy sink" or "energy cyst." Where previous trauma has occurred, subsequent injuries pool and are recorded over these original fascial injuries. In order to dissolve such an energy cyst, we need to match its energy and surpass it. In doing so, energy equilibrium can be restored.

The term *peizo-electric effect* refers to the ability of some materials to transform mechanical force into electrical energy. Percussion creates just enough energy to dissolve the energy-sink effect on damaged and restricted tissue and allows normal circuitry to be re-established with its normal flow and symmetry. The combination of the vibrational force of the motor speed of the percussor, the pressure applied by the monitoring hand, and the vectors between them yields the desired conditions for release.

The therapist must hold back the tissues with the monitoring hand to let enough energy buildup to surpass the quantity of energy from whatever injury that caused the fascial connective tissue deformation.

Dr. Fulford believed that intent was more important than technique. The physician's thoughts and intent need to be pure and focused. In biophysics, this makes sense on an electromagnetic level. Thoughts and living beings are both made up of electromagnetic energy. Your thoughts affect the field of people you touch.

Fulford believed that the hammer was an extension of the operator's pure thought to release the restriction or energy sink.

The purpose of the therapist's opposing or free hand is not to follow the unwinding tissue, but to resist its unwinding in order to allow a deep fascial release as the energy sink is freed. It's better to be on an area too short a period of time or with too soft a touch than too long or hard.

This release is sometimes very subtle, and many therapists don't feel it at first. It may take much practice with hands-on instruction. Science verifies that life, matter, existence and the brain waves of all thought are composed of vibrations or oscillating wavelengths and frequencies. The highest form of vibration is spirit, and the lowest is dense matter. Dr. Fulford believed the vibrations produced by the percussor helped to improve the vibratory rhythm of patients at all levels when directed by the vibrations of pure love and loving intent with its use.

THE NERVOUS SYSTEM AND BREATHING

The autonomic nervous system is influenced by fascial connective tissue restrictions and can be balanced by fascial release. The actual emotional feeling of the trauma or event is usually stored in the fascia; however, the memory of the feeling is thought to be in the brain. The brain will influence the flow of the Craniosacral Fluid (CSF).

As you see, the body can't be separated into parts, as it's all interconnected through the fascia and the energy field of the body. Breathing is the most elementary of our body's functions and can be involuntary or voluntary, conscious or unconscious. Breathing is a major link between our mind and body. The CSF is pumped by our craniosacral movement, which should follow a harmonious pumping pattern just as our breathing rhythms should be balanced and full. Unbalanced breathing affects the sleep cycle and can cause mental disturbances.

TOXIC ELIMINATION AND BREATHING

Our elimination system needs to be fully operational for optimal health. Only 10% of our wastes are eliminated by the bowel and urine; another 20% is eliminated by the skin, and 70% by breathing and exhaled water vapor. So, it's clear that if you improve your breathing, you can improve your overall health. We recommend specific breathing exercises and techniques to free the breath with the Percussor, Adjustor and the Erchonia Laser.

● ●

A Case History of Hiatal Hernia

I was referred by Dr. Stephan B., DO, to Brimhall Chiropractic Clinic for a hiatal hernia. I was experiencing back pain, stomach pain and chest pain. After the first treatment, the hiatal hernia stopped bothering me and the stomach pain was gone. After the physical changes began and my health changed, the depression I experienced changed and my whole outlook on life brightened. I think every part of my body was worked on from the cranium to my toes; with acupuncture on scar tissue, deep muscle massage, the laser, the cleansing baths and the supplements that helped me to regain my health. If anyone wants to change his or her quality of life, I would strongly suggest going through the program at the Brimhall Wellness Center.

— Enid F.

● ●

SUMMARY

- We don't treat conditions that have people; we treat people who have conditions.
- We live in a body that knows how to take care of itself if it is not interfered with.
- The task of the doctor is not to treat conditions, but to re-establish the structural integrity of the body.
- Each part of the cranium, spine, nervous system and fascia can affect any and every part of the body.
- 3 groundbreaking tools for re-establishing structural integrity are:

  1. The Erchonia Adjustor
  2. Cold Laser
  3. Percussor

Adjustor   Percussor   Laser

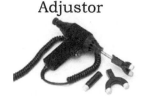 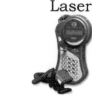

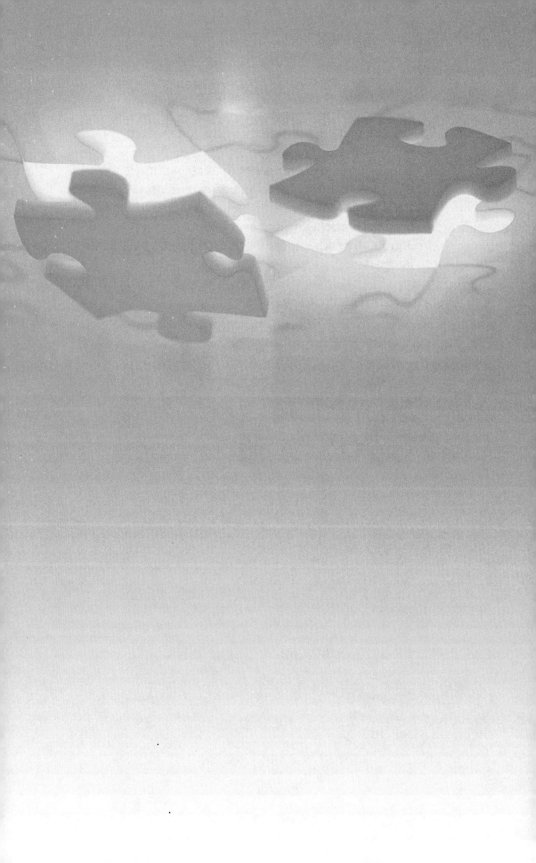

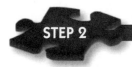

REBALANCE ELECTROMAGNETICS

ELECTROMAGNETIC POLLUTION

Our bodies are synchronized with the natural rhythms of the earth, moon and sun. When this field is interfered with, we get sick. Unfortunately, because of modern technological advances, we now live in a sea of electromagnetism. Abnormal electromagnetism, TVs, radios, computers, electric appliances and power lines surround us, constantly emitting electromagnetic signals.

As electromagnetic pollution accumulates, our glands become stressed to the point of exhaustion, our vision declines and our cells no longer know how to build and repair the body properly. Electromagnetic pollution puts the body in an alarm state and robs the body of zinc and other nutrients.

IS THERE AN "ELECTROPOLLUTION" SOLUTION?

Much of this electromagnetic pollution or "electropollution" can be avoided. The rest can be rebalanced. The brain's healthiest rhythms can be put back into proper alignment. So, even though we can't avoid the electromagnetic pollution in our environment, we fortunately have the technology to help protect ourselves.

THE EARTH'S ELECTROMAGNETIC FIELD

To understand electropollution, you must first know about our earth's electromagnetic field. The spinning molten iron core of Earth generates a gigantic magnetic field surrounding the planet. The sun gives off a constant solar wind of atomic particles that interact with the Earth's magnetic field, creating a protective magnetosphere that shields the Earth from damaging radiation. The interactions of the Earth's magnetic field and the sun's solar winds produce a constantly oscillating magnetic field of rising and falling waves.

Our daily biological rhythms are synchronized with these magnetic waves. The Earth, in its pristine state, would have provided humankind with better physical conditions for optimal health.

The Earth is a giant magnet with north and south poles, which only several decades ago generated a magnetic strength of 4 gauss (a unit of magnetic strength). Now the earth's magnetic field in most areas is said to have declined to only one-half gauss. Although this may be a part of a natural cycle taking place over years of geologic time, it's feared that this steady decline in magnetic field strength is the result of human intervention. Some say it may be caused by the loss of ozone.

Humans produce a field of 1 gauss. That means that when we're walking on the earth, which is at only one-half gauss, we're being drained.

Human-created electromagnetic fields <u>do</u> produce health hazards. Electric power transmission lines carry power that produces an electromagnetic field between 50 Hz and 60 Hz (50 to 60 cycles per second) – cycles that aren't present in the natural magnetic spectrum of Earth. Microwaves operate between billions and trillions of times per second. The highest naturally occurring frequency is way below our artificially created ones at 30 Hz.

The growth of electric power and communications systems has increased 5 to 10% per year since World War II. Telephone and satellite transmission systems now flood the Earth with radar and microwave transmissions from 25,000 miles out in space. Receiving stations for radio, TV and cellular phones are becoming ubiquitous. Electrical power transmission uses millions of volts and thousands of amperes, while military systems use all parts of the electromagnetic spectrum for communication, surveillance and weaponry.

Every transmitting and receiving device produces an electromagnetic field. As we listen to the radio, watch TV or answer the cell phone, our bodies are being bombarded by the same energy transmitted by radio, TV stations and shortwave transmitters. We're placed in a sewer of abnormal electromagnetic pollution by the very things that make our lives convenient --

- TVs
- Cell phones
- Radar devices
- Electric power transmission lines
- Lighting fixtures

- Home appliances
- Electric ovens
- Microwave ovens
- Toasters
- Hair dryers

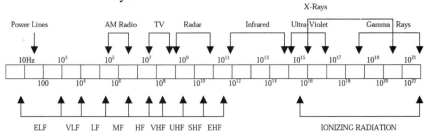

HOW "ELECTROPOLLUTION" STARTED MAKING US SICK

Some of the earliest warnings about electromagnetic fields surfaced in 1928. The General Electric Plant in Schenectady, New York, was in the process of building a radio transmitter that produced the highest frequency possible at that time, 27 megahertz. The workers at the plant complained of feeling vaguely ill. Medical investigation revealed that the workers experienced a two-degree elevation of temperature, accompanied by other symptoms such as sweating, weakness, nausea and dizziness – all within 15 minutes of exposure to this field.

During World War II, radar was invented. In 1942, U.S. Navy personnel recorded the same kind of symptoms associated with the rise in body temperature identified earlier. Other 1940s studies, with workers at blast furnaces and animal models studying the same environment, found that the thermal and non-thermal effects of microwave radiation produced early signs of cataract formation after only three days of exposure. These became known as microwave cataracts.

The first factory studies in Sweden showed that factories testing microwave equipment had workers with significant incidence of cataracts and nerve damage to the retina.

Other factories, such as the Hughes Aircraft Corp. in 1953, reported bleeding tendencies, higher incidence of leukemia and brain tumors among its workers. Experimental studies with plants at the time reported chromosomal damage to garlic plants exposed to microwave radiation.

In the 1980's, an experiment with animal models finally identified many of the effects of microwave radiation. The first effect of microwave radiation is stress, indicated biochemically by an increase in stress hormones, plasma cortisol and triglycerides. The animals in the study grew cancers in the glands associated with stress and stress exhaustion: the adrenal, thyroid and pituitary.

Other animal experiments demonstrated genetic consequences of microwave exposure: lower sperm count, sperm abnormalities and an increase in fetal death.

• • • • • • • • • • • • • • • • • • • •

Microwaves and Birth Defects

Hospital surveys of 69,277 human infants suggested that 30% of birth defects are not the result of family history, but of external causes. Mount Vernon, New Jersey, ranks fifth in the nation for the numbers of microwave transmitters in use. Furthermore, the incidence of Down's Syndrome in the same location is 1,000% above the national average.

• •

The evidence that artificially produced electromagnetic fields promote cancer is clearly suggested, partly by the effect of genetic mutation and partly by the effect of accelerated cell growth associated with cancer.

British studies indicated that people who lived near electric power lines had a higher incidence of mental disturbances and suicides.

In rat studies, 60 Hz fields produced lower learning rates with greater numbers of mistakes. In studies with monkeys, three weeks of exposure to such fields immediately depressed serotonin and dopamine levels in the spinal fluid, an effect lasting for several months after the exposure. Both of these neurotransmitters are involved in behavioral and psychological mechanisms and could account for mental disturbances.

Other animal studies found reduction in melatonin levels (melatonin is associated with healthful, restorative sleep), as well as testosterone reductions and birth defects. Dairy farmers have reported declines in production of milk from cows after high-power lines are installed close to herds.

All artificially made electromagnetic fields from microwave, radio wave and alternating current – regardless of frequency – produce health hazards in varying degrees.

REVERT TO THE STONE AGE?

Should you throw away all your electronically based conveniences? No, of course not! But you can live more healthfully by protecting yourself from their transmissions. Here are a few ideas.

LOCATION, LOCATION, LOCATION

Location affects the strength of the ambient electromagnetic fields we live in. Studies show that suburban homes have a 1 to 3 milligauss field strength (a measure of ambient electromagnetic pollution), while rural homes show strengths of generally less than 1 milligauss. Field intensities greater than 3 milligauss are related to a higher incidence of cancer and other physiological and mental disorders, so the location of your home can have a direct impact on your health.

The intensity of the electropollution can be also increased many times by hazards such as –

- Workplace environments filled with computers and electronic equipment
- Living within 100 yards of a broadcast tower
- Living close to power lines

We can reduce the amount of our daily exposure by taking a few simple steps.

DON'T SIT SO CLOSE TO THE TV!

Our mothers were right. Sitting too close to the TV is bad for us. Newer TVs and computers give off less intense electromagnetic fields than older models, and the size of the screen determines the amount of power and the corresponding field that the TV produces. For instance, a 13-inch screen TV produces a 1-milligauss field of about 40 inches in all directions (it varies a bit by manufacturer). Sitting beyond this field (allowing more space for larger TVs) places you in a safe position. Manufacturers suggest sitting no closer than 5 feet as a general rule.

• •

Yes, TV Is Bad for You

TVs and computers give off radiation fields in all directions, not just in front of the screen. A child's bed should never be placed against a wall opposite a TV set.

• •

COMPUTERS AND RADIATION

A recent study reported that people working with computers more than 20 hours per week have a higher incidence of birth defects, cataracts, eye strain, disturbance in menstrual cycles, skin rashes and a cluster of symptoms linked with chronic stress, such as fatigue, headache, sleep disturbances and nausea. Although the radiation from computers extends as far away as a half mile, sitting back at least 30 inches from the screen will reduce the strength of the radiation to less than 1 milligauss. Moving the keyboard back and wearing corrective lenses can be a partial solution to this electropollution.

THE HAZARDS OF FLUORESCENT LIGHTS

Fluorescent lights produce a host of problems caused by the electromagnetic spectrum of color. Most of the problems are associated with the cheapest pink-tinted lights. There are lesser problems reported from use of the more expensive blue-tinted fixtures, and very few problems when full-spectrum light is used, according to the work of John Ott. Pink-tinted fluorescents are associated with irritability and aggressive behavior when people are exposed to more than three hours of this lighting.

Fluorescents are safe beyond a distance of one foot. Thus, they shouldn't be used as floor or desk lamps because of their proximity to the user. Incandescent light is much closer to sunlight and only produces a 60 Hz field of 0.05 milligauss at 6 inches. When possible, choose incandescent lights, and turn off fluorescent lights.

CLOCKS

Electric clocks are safe if placed 2 feet away from the user, especially during periods of long exposure such as sleep. Battery-operated clocks produce a negligible field and are safer alternatives to electric clocks.

MICROWAVES

While the microwave is operating, don't stand in front of it. Of course, microwaving destroys nutrients like folic acid, alters nutrients in a way that makes you fat, and microwaved food has shown traces of radiation, so you won't be microwaving anyway, right?

CORDLESS AND CELL PHONES

The hazards of personal radio transmitters, cell phones and cordless phones increase with length of use. Use them as little as possible and for the shortest duration possible.

• •

KINESIOLOGY SELF-TEST

If you feel weak, have headaches or just feel generally ill when you work in front of computers or under fluorescent lights, it may be caused by electromagnetic pollution.

Try this simple test using kinesiology. Stand and put your arm straight out in front of you when you are several feet away from any electric appliance. Have someone push down on your arm and see how strong it is. This gives you a baseline for comparison. Then, turn on a hand-held hair dryer and hold it next to your body (or stand within 30 inches of a computer screen or within 2 feet of a TV that is turned on) and test the same arm for strength. You'll probably find your arm becomes completely weak close to the electric appliance.

Next, hold a bottle of Nutri-West plant-derived digestive enzymes (such as Total Enzymes™) and retest your arm within the same electromagnetic field. Your arm will strengthen. Why? Everything has electromagnetic energy. Some things weaken us, others strengthen us. Natural plant enzymes are one supplement that will help protect you from electromagnetic pollution.

Synergistic nutrients that support the adrenals like the one we use, DSF™ (de-stress formula), do the same thing. If you took a picture of your blood on Darkfield (live blood analysis) exam before taking adrenal support or before taking the plant enzymes, you would frequently see sticky blood cells. Within minutes of chewing a living enzyme or the DSF supplement, you would see the blood cells lose their stickiness and begin to move more freely. This is the effect of the positive electromagnetic field from the living food affecting your blood.

Why do adrenal nutrients work? Electromagnetic stress depletes the adrenal system. Your body will tell you if you need adrenal support.

Kinesiology or muscle response testing is a way of communicating with the body. Things that are good for you will make you strong, and those that aren't, make you weak. It's the body's way of talking to you. Living foods and nutritional support give a boost to your electromagnetics, one of your defense systems.

• •

SOME ELECTROMAGNETIC FIELDS ARE GOOD

Robert O. Becker, MD, showed some electromagnetic fields produced by direct current (DC) batteries were actually beneficial, accelerating bone-healing success rates by 80%. The human body itself is a DC organism.

The potentially harmful electromagnetic fields set up by alternating currents, electric power lines outside the home, transmission lines in the home and fields generated by our everyday electrical appliances, can interfere with our own DC energy field, nervous system and health.

HEALING WITH MAGNETS

Even though we can't (and wouldn't) want to do away with all our electric appliances, we can protect ourselves. A simple multi-polar magnet, no bigger than a credit card, can energize your energy field and protect you. This small multi-polar magnet can be placed in a shirt pocket,

Multi-Polar Magnets
www.brimhall.com

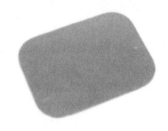

inside a woman's bra or in a wallet carried on the body. We use very specific magnets that change from north to south on the same side, four to five times per inch, and they're under 350 gauss no matter where you measure them.

We recommend people wear this magnet all the time they are working with computers or around other strong electromagnetic environments. Our preference is to wear it all day long, every day. Why? Electromagnetic pollution is everywhere and is most likely affecting you. Usually people have more energy and feel better when they have this very specific magnet next to them.

Multi-polar magnets may also be used for pain reduction by placing them over the painful area and leaving it until the pain lessens or leaves. If this doesn't help or makes it worse, move it to the exact same location on the opposite side of the body. This effect has to do with activating the acupuncture or energy meridians of the body. This credit-card-sized magnet can increase circulation and relieve chronic pain including –

- Headaches
- Carpal tunnel syndrome
- Aches and pains
- Tennis elbow
- Strained muscle problems
- Bruises
- Arthritis
- Old injuries
- Back pain or spinal problems due to the balancing of energy

Most people wear the multi-polar magnet all day. Some feel they need more energy and find that placing several under their mattress pad of their beds helps them at night. You can order them from Brimhall Wellness Seminars at 866-338-4883 or www.brimhall. com

LARGE-SCALE ELECTROMAGNETIC PROTECTION

Certain equipment has been developed to protect our magnetic field, thus helping neutralize harmful electromagnetic fields of radiation.

The sluggishness, fatigue, nausea, dizziness, irritability, eye strain, rashes and other health problems associated with continuous exposure to high electromagnetic fields (above 30 Hz) can be counteracted with a device designed to blanket an area of about 20,000 square feet. This larger unit was designed to protect a home or office environment against harmful grid lines, geomagnetic disturbances, artificially generated electromagnetic standing waves, extremely low frequencies (ELF frequencies) and other harmful waves.

TOTAL SHIELD

We highly recommend a device called Total Shield, which is composed of two separate electronic generators. One generator is a detector device that identifies the frequencies of the geomagnetic disturbances and grid lines from the environment and broadcasts them back out through a Tesla coil, which cancels out the disturbance.

The other generator is a 7.83 frequency generator, which duplicates the Schumann resonance (the resonant frequency of the Earth's magnetic field).

Normally, one of these units is sufficient to protect a large home or office area. However, where electromagnetic pollution is severe, such as areas near high-voltage power lines, transmitting towers for TV or radio towers, more than one unit might be necessary to overcome the severity of the pollution.

According to some electrical engineers, the Total Shield unit will also strip radiation pollution from your body.

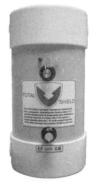

Total Shield
www.brimhall.com

Total Shield Success Stories

After having Total Shield up and running for about a week, I am decidedly less fatigued now from working long hours at the computer. The difference is striking. Before, I felt debilitated. Now, that sensation has disappeared. I also got some effect with respect to the TV. I could habitually take no more than one hour of TV watching without feeling worn down ... but the other evening, I spent nearly three hours in front of the idiot box without ill effect.

—A resident of Paris, France

After using Total Shield, a dairyman reported that his cows' milk production had risen and the percentage of cream in his milk had dramatically increased.

REGAIN PERFECT HARMONY

Electropollution can interfere, jam or alter brainwave patterns, cellular communication, sleep cycles and circadian rhythms. Symptoms caused by the depletion of our environment (what is now called Magnetic Deficiency Syndrome) include:

- Stiffness in the shoulders, back and neck
- Lumbago
- Chest pains
- Headaches
- Dizziness
- Insomnia
- Hypertension
- Digestive disorders
- Bone and nerve diseases

The Earth's natural magnetic resonance is created in a constant interaction between the Earth's surface, the atmosphere, the ionosphere and the radiation of the sun. The dynamics of this interaction create discharge effects, including the occurrence of electrical fields of charged particles that are discharged by lightning strikes and an electromagnetic field that pulses at an average of 7.83 cycles per second (the Schumann resonance).

This 7.83 frequency function is believed to be the coordinating signal for healthy life on the planet. All life is bioelectrical as well as biochemical. When our bioelectrical system is altered by pollution, our biochemical system will be affected in some way.

The Earth resonance of 7.83 Hz falls into the alpha brainwave frequency, which helps synchronize our brainwaves with its most relaxed and alert state.

THE MINI HARMONIZER

A device called The Mini Harmonizer is a good tool for achieving emotional, mental and physical harmony in an abnormal electromagnetic and stressful environment. It helps balance your immediate environment within electromagnetic "smog," offers biofeedback entrainment to alpha and theta brainwave states for stress relief, and helps rebalance bodily energy flow.

The Mini Harmonizer first supplies your environment with a stable, earthlike magnetic field at the natural Schumann resonance of 7.83 cycles per second. The Mini Harmonizer helps keep a balanced electromagnetic field.

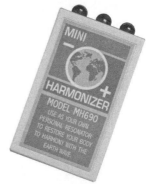

Mini Harmonizer

www.brimhall.com

On the top of the Mini Harmonizer are three large, flashing lights that can be used for a quick, effective biofeedback session whenever needed. As you look at the lights, a process called entrainment takes place and you experience the peaceful awareness and calming effects associated with the alpha states. One switch on the side of the tool allows you to set the unit to this 7.83 Hz frequency, or you can set it to 3.91 Hz, the theta position.

The 7.83 setting represents a state of conscious, relaxed awareness and enhanced creativity. The 3.91 theta setting has a deeper, more profoundly relaxing effect than the alpha setting and is close to the normal brainwave pattern of a person before he or she enters sleep. We teach patients how to use this instrument to complement their health.

SUMMARY

- Our bodies are synchronized with the natural rhythms of the earth, moon and sun. When this field is interfered with, we get sick.
- All artificially made electromagnetic fields from microwave, radio wave and alternating current – regardless of frequency – produce health hazards in varying degrees.
- A simple multi-polar magnet, no bigger than a credit card, can energize your energy field and protect you.
- Total Shield can protect a large home or office area from harmful electromagnetic waves.
- The Mini Harmonizer is a good tool for achieving emotional, mental and physical harmony in an abnormal electromagnetic and stressful environment.

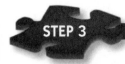

REBUILD WITH NUTRITION: THE BODY AS A COMPUTER

Step 3A
Reset Adrenals and the General Adaptive Syndrome (GAS)

A) Reset Adrenals and The General Adaptive System
B) Replenish Nutrition for Organ, Glands or System Weakness
C) Reduce Infective Organisms in the Body
D) Replace Enzymes and/or HCL to Aid Digestion, Assimilation and Elimination
E) Restore Proper Bowel Flora to Optimize Colon Function

Your adrenals are the small glands above each kidney that produce hormones. They must work well for the rest of the body to heal. Unfortunately, under stress, the adrenals don't work well, potentially causing disease in the body.

Dr. Hans Selye, in his book *Stress Without Distress*, demonstrated the effects of stress on glands in the body. His work clarified a General Adaptive Syndrome (GAS), which describes the body's short - and long-term reaction to stress.

Dr. Selye found that excessive work, play or emotional upset would cause exactly the same reaction: the adrenal cortex hypertrophies – that is, it becomes enlarged due to growth in cell size. (Hypertrophy can be thought of as the opposite of the more commonly known condition, atrophy).

While the adrenal cortex grows in this condition, the thymus gland and the lymph nodes shrink, compromising the immune system. These effects take place simultaneously and are accompanied by stomach and intestinal irritation and ulceration.

The 3 Stages of GAS
1. The alarm reaction
2. The stage of resistance
3. The stage of exhaustion

DE-STRESSING WITH GLANDULAR NUTRITION OR HERBS

We use "glandulars" to help jump-start the adrenals and other systems of the body. Glandulars are freeze-dried tablets containing defatted glands, organs or other tissues from cow or pork sources. We have also formulated Herbal DSF (de-stress formula) for vegetarians. They've long been used to provide whole gland nutrition to support the healthy and proper functioning of glands.

Glandulars help restore normal activity to glands that are damaged, deteriorated or attacked by the autoimmune system. The roots of glandular therapy can be traced to early in the 20th century, when Dr. Royal Lee found whole-gland nutrition had special biochemical agents that helped start the repair process.

Glandulars help reverse and "reset" these stressed glands so they begin to function normally. We have found if you don't de-stress the person with this nutritional support, they do not respond to other treatment effectively. In fact, the body is neurologically confused, or what we refer to as "switched." When the body is switched, it does not give proper information, nor can it heal properly. The patient might even react opposite to a prescribed drug or nutrition. For instance, Vitamin C may give them a cold, or a drug to lower blood pressure may actually raise it. Other nutrients may seem to irritate the gastrointestinal tract or cause the opposite of the desired effect.

TRACE MINERALS

It's important that the trace minerals zinc, iodine and chromium accompany the glandulars and herbals to promote necessary enzymatic activity, because enzymes are the building blocks of our existence. They are co-factors or helpers to proper chemical actions.

If you experience a drop in blood pressure (maybe even get

dizzy) when you stand from a seated or recumbent position, it's a sign your adrenals are under stress. If your pupils dilate when light is shined on them, you have another sign of overstressed adrenals. (When you're healthy, your pupils should contract in the presence of light.) Specific lab tests from saliva or urine can confirm these findings.

Stabilizing blood sugar with adrenal malfunction can be difficult, manifesting symptoms of hyper- or hypoglycemic symptoms.

To restate our findings: in a severe GAS condition, every system may respond poorly, or in reverse, to what's expected. A person subject to this condition won't give coherent structural, nutritional or emotional signals to the practitioner nor respond properly to treatment.

We've found the best way to begin the healing process is to have people chew the De-Stress (DSF) nutrients. After chewing, most patients show the beginnings of a rapid improvement on both physical and emotional levels. This is an oversimplification of the whole-health process, of course, and is only the beginning of total, proper care.

• • • • • • • • • • • • • • • • • • • •

One Case History

A few years ago, a man came in with a positive disc and was recommended for surgery. He opted for us to do conservative structural treatment instead. Treatment went well and he became stable with only periodic structural "tune-ups," as he called them. But then he was promoted to a supervisory job with new emotional stress. To offset the stress, he played racquetball. This was okay until a younger player challenged him. Now he added physical stressors to his emotional ones.

All stresses are interpreted by the body and accumulated. An *alarm* state leads to *resistance,* and then to *exhaustion.* He then became what we call "symptomatic expressive." A person's weakest link will usually be the first to show a symptom.

In this man's case, it was his back. He came into the office almost crawling. We had to reset his adrenals nutritionally and then correct the structural imbalance to allow him the health and wellness he sought.

· ●

· ·

Stress Can Lead to:

- Bad Digestion
- Insomnia
- Memory Loss
- Decreased Sexual Drive/Ability
- Increased Cortisol and Weight Gain (Syndrome X)
- Rapid Heart Beat
- High Blood Pressure
- Susceptibility to Infections
- Exaggeration of Allergies
- Arthritis or other Connective Tissue Conditions
- Back Problems
- Skin Disorders
- Anxiety
- Irritability
- Depression

· ●

THE DANGERS OF STRESS

Nearly 80% of all health problems are stress-related. Lack of sleep, overwork, illness, excessive alcohol consumption and smoking are common physical causes of stress. Emotional pressures of deadlines, life changes, birth, death, marriage, divorce, holidays, noise, temperature extremes, and temperature changes can all put stress on the body.

There are specific energy points on the body that can reflect system or organ stress. A Brimhall Wellness practitioner would use this total person scan, with muscle response testing, as one part of this evaluation.

Other testing that might be accomplished could be case history, physical exam, questionnaire, hair and blood analysis, computerized electrodermal testing, etc.

Chart I – Primary Reflexes

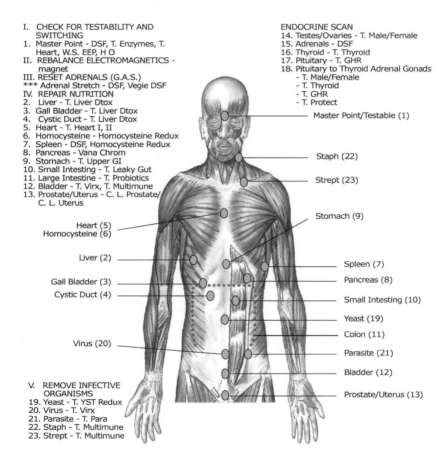

I. CHECK FOR TESTABILITY AND SWITCHING
1. Master Point - DSF, T. Enzymes, T. Heart, W.S. EEP, H O
II. REBALANCE ELECTROMAGNETICS - magnet
III. RESET ADRENALS (G.A.S.)
*** Adrenal Stretch - DSF, Vegie DSF
IV. REPAIR NUTRITION
2. Liver - T. Liver Dtox
3. Gall Bladder - T. Liver Dtox
4. Cystic Duct - T. Liver Dtox
5. Heart - T. Heart I, II
6. Homocysteine - Homocysteine Redux
7. Spleen - DSF, Homocysteine Redux
8. Pancreas - Vana Chrom
9. Stomach - T. Upper GI
10. Small Intesting - T. Leaky Gut
11. Large Intestine - T. Probiotics
12. Bladder - T. Virx, T. Multimune
13. Prostate/Uterus - C. L. Prostate/ C. L. Uterus

ENDOCRINE SCAN
14. Testes/Ovaries - T. Male/Female
15. Adrenals - DSF
16. Thyroid - T. Thyroid
17. Pituitary - T. GHR
18. Pituitary to Thyroid Adrenal Gonads
   - T. Male/Female
   - T. Thyroid
   - T. GHR
   - T. Protect

Master Point/Testable (1)

Staph (22)

Strept (23)

Stomach (9)

Heart (5)
Homocysteine (6)

Liver (2)

Gall Bladder (3)

Cystic Duct (4)

Spleen (7)

Pancreas (8)

Small Intesting (10)

Yeast (19)

Colon (11)

Virus (20)

Parasite (21)

Bladder (12)

V. REMOVE INFECTIVE ORGANISMS
19. Yeast - T. YST Redux
20. Virus - T. Virx
21. Parasite - T. Para
22. Staph - T. Multimune
23. Strept - T. Multimune

Prostate/Uterus (13)

Chart II – Secondary Reflexes

Bladder = T. Virx, T. Multimune

Blood Pressure = T. Heart I,II, Homocysteine Redux

Blood Vitality = Homocysteine Redux, Hemo Lyph

Brain = T. Brain, C.L. Brain-Spinal, C.L. RNA

Colon = T. Probiotics, T. L-Glutamine

Fluid Retention = T. Heart I,II

Ileocecal Valve = T. Probiotics, T. L-Glutamine

Kidney = T. Chelate, C.L. Kidney

Lung = T. Virx, T. Multimune, C.L. Lung

Master Point = DSF, Enzymes, H20, T. Heart

Non-Infectious Allergies = T. Liver, T. System Dtox

Ovary = T. GHR, T. Female, C.L. Ovary

Parathyroid = T. Calcium, T. GHR

Primary Hormone = T. GHR, T. Male/Female

Prostate = C.L. Prostate, Prostate Health

Testicle = T. GHR, C.L. Orchid, T. Male

Thyroid = T. Thyroid, T. GHR, C.L. Thyroid

Toxin = T. Liver Dtox, T. System Dtox

Uterus = C.L. Uterus

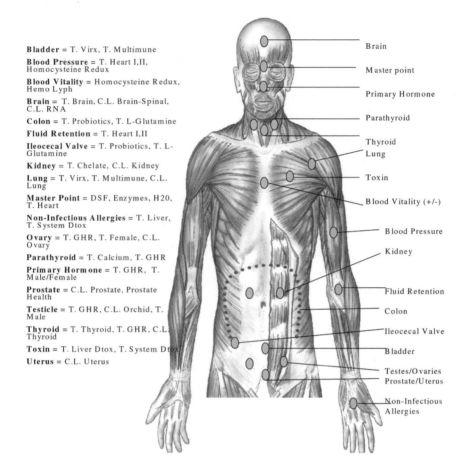

Brain

Master point

Primary Hormone

Parathyroid

Thyroid
Lung

Toxin

Blood Vitality (+/-)

Blood Pressure

Kidney

Fluid Retention

Colon

Ileocecal Valve

Bladder

Testes/Ovaries
Prostate/Uterus

Non-Infectious
Allergies

SUMMARY

- Increased demands on the adrenal glands are responsible for the common conditions associated with stress, called the General Adaptation Syndrome (GAS).
- Chronic stress depletes the immune system, which leads to illness, hormonal imbalances in adrenals, thymus and other glands.
- "Glandulars," herbs and trace minerals help jump-start the adrenals and other systems of the body.
- Degenerative disease and overall poor health may get its start with adrenal exhaustion and the GAS.

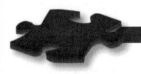

Step 3B
Replenish Nutrition for Organ, Glands or System Weakness

Population surveys show that 20% of Americans never eat vegetables, and 40% rarely consume fruit or fruit juices. Another 80% never consume whole grains or high-fiber foods.

The most popular vegetable consumed in the U.S. is the potato, but usually in the non-nutritious forms of French fries and potato chips.

It's clear that the standard American diet, which is high in sugar and low in fruits and vegetables, has left Americans deficient in many nutrients.

5-A-DAY FRUITS AND VEGETABLES

Fruit and vegetable consumption has been consistently shown to reduce the risk of such degenerative diseases as diabetes, heart disease and cancer. The "5-a-day for Better Health" program sponsored by the National Cancer Institute (NCI) encourages the public to include at least five servings of fruits and vegetables in their daily diet.

SUGAR'S NOT SO SWEET

Sugar is used as a flavor and texture enhancer in nearly all processed and fast foods, adding hundreds of empty calories and depleting the body of nutrients.

All forms of refined sugar lower immune system function by interfering with the abilities of white blood cells to destroy unfriendly bacteria. Alcohol, a sugar relative, weakens a wide variety of immune responses.

WE'RE FEEDING ON CHEMICALS INSTEAD OF NUTRITION

With depleted soil robbing our food of nutrition, and diets high in sodium, protein, sugar, soft drinks, caffeine and processed foods, we're suffering from mineral and nutritional deficiency like never before.

And, if that weren't enough, the chemicals in our food system are overwhelming our body systems. An estimated 15% of the U.S. population suffers from fatigue associated with Multiple Chemical Sensitivities. The EPA has identified over 400 toxic chemicals in human tissue associated with fatigue, depression, mental, motor, neurological disorders and cancer.

WHAT'S THE SOLUTION?

Avoid empty foods to stop depleting your body. Choose fresh foods over canned food. Drink 8-10 glasses of pure water to assist with toxin removal. Rebuild the body and immune system with natural whole foods and good supplements. When the body's systems are working at 100%, you enjoy 100% health.

• • • • • • • • • • • • • • • • • • •

Kinesiology: The Body's Language

A wide variety of diagnostic tools can be used to identify organs and body systems that may be under stress. Blockages in the vertebrae of the spinal cord and related structural stress patterns are indicators that the switches your body uses to heal itself are turned off. The structure of your body rules its functions, so the foundation must be rebuilt.

Each organ or system that can be identified as "under stress" can be supported by nutrition and structural support. Muscle response testing, or kinesiology, is the body's way of talking to you and telling you what's going on.

• •

LIVER AND GALLBLADDER

The liver is the largest organ in the body by weight. Digested food is brought to the liver by the blood. It plays an important role in the body's metabolism and use of carbohydrates, fats and proteins. The liver produces bile, which is sent to the gallbladder for storage and use by the duodenum in digestion of fats. It also produces blood-clotting substances, important for wound repair and anti-blood-clotting substances, to help keep the blood system clear.

The liver regulates blood sugar, detoxifies the body, produces Vitamin A from dietary sources and acts as a storage depot for Vitamin A, fat, Vitamin B12, Vitamin D and Vitamin K.

When the liver is overloaded by too many body wastes, infectious organisms and toxins from the environment, it loses its ability to protect the body. The typical American diet can be damaging to the liver, resulting in allergies, digestive problems and an inability to detoxify harmful substances.

The gallbladder is a pear-shaped sac located beneath the right lobe of the liver. It stores and releases bile produced in the liver, which is important in aiding the digestion of fat. The gallbladder also plays other important roles with fatty acids and the movement of food through the GI tract.

If you awaken every morning between 1-3 a.m., in acupuncture understanding, that may be a sign that your liver needs attention. If the liver or gallbladder is identified as being under stress from any source, there are powerful protective nutrients that can help strengthen and rebuild their tissues.

Total Liver D-Tox™

A total complex nutrition we developed called Total Liver D-Tox™ contains many of the synergistic nutrient supports for replenishing the liver and gallbladder.

THE HEART

Your heart is about the size of your fist and weighs less than a pound. It's a hollow, mostly muscular organ that beats 72 times per minute at rest. That adds up to at least 104,000 beats per day and 38 million beats in a year. It's been estimated that the heart pumps enough blood in one week to fill a swimming pool!

Besides being a mechanical pump for blood, the heart's also a generator of electricity. In a way similar to the power that is generated as water flows over a dam, electricity is generated in the body as the heart pumps blood through the arteries. The heart is the largest generator of electricity in the body and, therefore, controls the functions of the brain. It generates about two-and-a-half watts with each contraction.

"The arteries are supreme," said Andrew Taylor Still, the founder of osteopathy. He felt that communication existed for the whole body through the arterial blood system. Science now acknowledges that Still was correct and that the heart is our emotional center, just as our folklore and scripture recorded. For a deeper probe into the mysteries of the heart, *The Heart's Code*, by Dr. Paul Pearsal is a wonderful journey.

Heart disease is the number one cause of death in the United States. Americans suffer more than 1.5 million heart attacks each year, and more than one third die on their first attack. For half of the victims, the attack is their first warning signal that their heart's in trouble.

Although heart disease causes over 40% of all deaths and is responsible for over 550,000 heart attack deaths and 500,000 strokes each year, in the U.S. alone, heart disease is one of the most preventable of chronic conditions. By conservative estimates, more than 56,000 deaths each year could be prevented by identifying patients with high homocysteine levels and treating them with simple B vitamin supplements, according to recent research. Dietary changes, nutritional supplements, stress reduction and exercise can all lead to healthy arteries and a healthy heart.

Stresses from many sources contribute to the free radicals and toxins that oxidize cholesterol and cause heart problems. Those sources include excess homocysteine levels, oral contraceptives (which raise homocysteine), toxins from infectious diseases, chlorine

100

and fluoride in water, pesticides, processed foods, smoking and the free radicals produced from the intense heat of cooking.

In heart disease, a cascade of events is believed to take place. First, nutritional deficiencies weaken arterial walls, making them less elastic and less adaptable to stress. Next, stressors cause small tears in arterial walls and the body releases white blood cells to repair tissue damage. Oxidized LDL cholesterol is then deposited at the sites of damage, triggering soft plaque formation. Finally, calcium is attracted to the site and solid plaque forms, hardening the arteries and eventually leading to arteriosclerosis, heart disease and strokes.

High cholesterol levels, themselves, may not be the problem they were first thought to be. Oxidized LDL cholesterol is now believed to be the major problem.

Current research has shown that by age 15, many Americans already have fatty streaks in their major blood vessels. By age 60, as much as 80% of Americans may have some degree of blockage in the coronary arteries that supply the heart with blood.

Typical symptoms of inadequate heart function are tingling or numbness of the extremities, pain in the chest, dyspnea or labored, difficult breathing, swelling of the extremities and general fatigue. When the heart isn't electric enough to keep up with the body's demands, it may give other signs of complications, seemingly not even related to the heart. Low sex drive, apathy or depression can also be signs of heart trouble. Chronic fatigue, due to a low heart electrical output, may also signal heart disease.

High blood pressure may be due to suboptimal heart function. There have been cases cited where nutrition for the heart brought patients out of comas.

● ● ● ● ● ● ● ● ● ● ● ● ● ● ● ● ● ● ● ●

A Case of Bypass Surgery

Dear Dr. Brimhall,

In 1979, I had a heart attack and surgery for three bypasses. In 1986, I had surgery for aorta valve and one bypass. In 1991, I had a balloon job that kept one artery of the original three open, but lost the other two. In 1995, I started seeking more help, as I was so tired all the time. I couldn't get out of bed by myself and had much difficulty turning over. Walking became a shuffle, and I walked very slowly with the aid of a cane. After a CAT scan by my doctor back home, I was told that I may have to have an operation before I went into a wheelchair. Well, Dr. Brimhall, your program has kept me out of that wheelchair, has me walking without a cane, getting out of chairs by myself and not feeling so tired.

— Bernard C.

ONE OF THE CULPRITS

Excess homocysteine has recently emerged as a major contributor to heart disease, affecting 42% of those with cerebrovascular disease, 28% with peripheral artery disease and 30% of those with coronary artery disease.

40% of heart attacks and strokes in the U.S. may be the result of elevated homocysteine levels. Individuals with cardiovascular disease have been found to have 30% higher homocysteine levels than their healthy counterparts.

Excess homocysteine can generate free radicals that oxidize LDL cholesterol, which leads to plaque formation in the arteries. While dangerously high homocysteine levels lead to death, they're the most easily preventable factor among people with coronary heart disease.

We have found that high homocysteine levels are much more dangerous to the body than just the heart and arteries. It may be a major factor causing MS in many people. Also, homocysteine can irritate the linings of the brain, the nerves, all organs and all systems.

The typical American diet leaves us deficient in the very nutrients that can prevent excess homocysteine from being produced. The American Heart Association recommends adequate intakes of vitamins B6, B12 and folic acid for individuals with a history of elevated homocysteine levels and heart disease.

We have formulated a synergistic nutritional support called Homocysteine Redux™, which contains the nutrient combinations to help reduce homocysteine.

VIRUS AND HEART DISEASE

Cocksaxie virus attacks heart muscle and can cause heart failure. Many patients with heart problems also have viral or other infections. Specific nutritional support can help the body's immune system eliminate infections. Avoiding sugars and hydrogenated fats are also important for heart health.

Total Virx™ (veg) contains many of the synergistic nutrients to help support the body in warding off viral infections.

LDL CHOLESTEROL AND ARTERIES

People with elevated cholesterol levels have a higher risk of developing atherosclerosis than people with low cholesterol levels. When deposits of cholesterol, fat and calcium form in the major arteries supplying the heart, blood flow to the heart can become restricted and trigger heart attacks. Most doctors believe that total cholesterol levels should stay under 200 mg/dl. The balance of "bad" LDL cholesterol to "good" HDL cholesterol is thought to be more important than total cholesterol.

Being overweight and having diabetes are other risk factors. Having Syndrome X increases the likelihood of heart disease. Feed your heart properly so it can perform properly:

- Minimize high fat intake from dairy and meat
- Avoid refined sugars and hydrogenated fats, especially margarine
- Limit alcohol intake
- Limit or eliminate coffee
- Eat smaller, more frequent meals with fish, vegetables, fruit and other high-fiber foods such as whole grains
- Supplement with specific synergistic nutrition

The Case of a Stroke Survivor

Dr. Brett Brimhall treated Chuck, a stroke survivor, who was unable to use his right arm and hand and unable to vocalize, due to tongue deviation. His medical doctor told him there was no hope for improvement. After using the Erchonia 635 nm on the area of the brain indicated and with proper nutrition, etc., Chuck was able to raise his arm for the first time in nine years. His tongue also came back straight in his mouth, allowing his verbal skills to improve. When he saw his MD the next time, he reached up and shook hands with the arm and hand that were, "never to work again."

THYROID

Hypothyroidism and hyperthyroid conditions affect an estimated seven to eight million people in the U.S. Undiagnosed thyroid problems can be behind many unidentified symptoms of fatigue, recurring illnesses and other non-responsive health problems. Frequently, blood tests of hormone levels are normal, but body temperature is abnormally low, indicating a thyroid problem.

Symptoms of Underproduction of Thyroid Hormones

Weight gain, fatigue, muscle weakness, cramps, appetite loss, slow heart rate, low body temperature, sensitivity to cold, hair loss, dry skin, constipation, slow speech, difficulties in concentration, depression, irritability, painful periods, drooping swollen eyes, bumps on eyelids, swollen face, increased allergies, recurrent infections, goiters and calcium metabolism problems are all symptoms of underproduction of thyroid hormones. This condition is often associated with Wilson's syndrome, physical and emotional stress and Hashimoto's disease.

. . . . ●

● ● ● ● ● ● ● ● ● ● ● ● ● ● ● ● . . . . .

Symptoms of Overproduction of Thyroid Hormones

Overproduction of thyroid hormones may cause symptoms such as, weight loss, fatigue, anxiety, rapid heartbeat, tremors, moist skin, excessive sweating, sensitivity to heat, bulging eyes, goiters, diarrhea, other gastrointestinal disturbances and chest pain. This condition is often called Graves' disease.

. . . . ●

The thyroid is the body's thermostat. It secretes two hormones that regulate body temperature, energy usage and metabolism. The thyroid affects all cells in the body, including the synthesis of RNA protein and oxygen consumption by cells, which affects overall metabolism. Thyroid function influences and is influenced by the pituitary, adrenals, parathyroid and sex glands – all of which work together.

Underactive thyroid conditions respond many times when supplemented with thyroid glandulars and nutrients that nourish the thyroid gland. Digestive disorders and malabsorption are known to play roles in thyroid disorders.

● ● ● ● ● ● ● ● ● ● ● ● ● ● . . . . . .

Fluoride & Chlorine

Fluoride in tap water and toothpastes, as well as chlorine in tap water, block iodine receptors in the thyroid gland. Sulfa and antihistamine drugs aggravate iodine uptake by the thyroid.

. . . . ●

THE BRAIN

Four million people in the U.S. suffer from Alzheimer's Disease. Anxiety disorders, from mild unease to intense panic and fear, affect 10 million people. Over 28% of Americans suffer from some kind of mental disorder severe enough to require treatment. Depression and anxiety are the most common emotional problems, and incidences among children, adolescents and the elderly are rapidly increasing.

Possible causes of poor mental health are: nutrient deficiencies and imbalances, hormone imbalances, food allergies and sensitivities, toxic metal buildup, poor handling of stress, poor absorption of nutrients, hypoglycemia, aspartame, alcohol, smoking, medications, immune system malfunction, brain chemistry imbalance, addiction and withdrawal, environmental causes and non-full spectrum lighting or only partial spectrum lighting.

Social ties, support groups, stress reduction, relaxation techniques, music, breathing exercises, nutritional supplements and dietary and environmental changes, are all things that can help to prevent mental health disorders and even restore healthy mental functions.

Total Brain™ (veg) is a nutrient we formulated as a synergistic blend containing many nutrients that support brain function.

PANCREAS AND BLOOD SUGAR

Over five million Americans are now being treated for diabetes, and another five million are estimated to have undetected adult-onset diabetes. Still another 20 million are believed to have impaired glucose metabolism that may eventually lead to diabetes.

The National Institute of Health reported that diabetic complications have become the third-leading cause of death in the U.S. and that millions have become blind because of undiagnosed diabetic problems.

Complications of diabetes include blindness, atherosclerosis, heart disease, stroke, nerve damage, kidney failure, gangrene, coma and death.

Genetic propensity, a poor diet, obesity and lack of exercise are believed to be major causes of the disease. Most people take in too many sugars and carbohydrates. This leads to increased insulin production, sugar craving and weight gain.

What we need is to take in more good-quality fats. Our nervous system, immune system, hormones and brain are made of fats! Diets that emphasize good-quality fats, complex carbohydrates, high fiber, fresh fruits and vegetables can help lower insulin requirements and normalize blood sugar levels. Exercise can also help produce positive insulin-like effects. Supplements that contain PABA, cysteine or high amounts of Vitamins B1, B3 and C may inactivate insulin, which can work against you.

Avoidance of alcohol and tobacco are essential in diabetes; tobacco use impairs circulation and can lead to kidney damage in diabetics.

• •

The Case of "Syndrome X"

Dear Docs and Staff:

There's a little group of symptoms known as Syndrome X, which is related to heart disease and insulin resistance. The profile consists of high triglycerides, borderline diabetes, borderline high blood pressure, borderline high cholesterol, low HDL and excess abdominal fat. That's me, a 43-year-old woman who looks dang sexy (I have it on good authority) and had no actual control insight for this situation, yet you all managed to do me right in three little days. Wow. Within two weeks of seeing you, my diastolic blood pressure has remained a fairly stable 80. My tachycardia seems to be very much under control for the first time in 25 years. My fasting blood glucose level is back to a very normal range, without use of the Glucophage, which my MD had recommended (hey, its only side-effect is death, but that rarely happens, so not to worry). I really feel like I've been given a new life. The Electric Acupuncture Diagnostic machine is the biggest non-human hero in this equation, as far as I'm concerned. I miss some of the foods you found me allergic to, but it's worth it ... I did not imagine that I was reacting to practically everything I was eating. Thank you, one and all, for a great gift and for your kind treatment of me.

— Patricia

• •

• •

Total Alpha Lipoic Acid™ (veg) contains the synergistic nutrients that support the pancreas.

Vana-Chrom™ (veg) contains many of the nutrients that support normal blood sugar.

• •

EYES: LENS AND CATARACTS

Cataracts are the number one cause of blindness worldwide and the leading cause of impaired vision and blindness in the United States. Cataract surgery has now become one of the most frequently performed operations in the United States.

A cataract is a condition where the lens of the eye thickens and becomes cloudy or opaque, resulting in the inability to focus and admit light normally. People who develop cataracts experience a painless, gradual loss of vision that can lead to blindness. Occasionally, when cataracts swell, they can be causes of secondary glaucoma.

The most common form of cataract is the 'senile cataract,' which affects people over 65 years of age. It is believed to be caused by free radical damage from ultraviolet light, infrared light, fluorescent lighting, low-level radiation, the process of aging, diabetes, heavy metal poisoning, injury to the eye, free radicals in water and food, fried and processed foods. Other possible causes include the use of many drugs, (including tetracycline, steroidal drugs, oral contraceptives and antihistamines) reduced gastrointestinal absorption and uptake of nutrients.

Free radicals can damage structural proteins, enzymes and cell membranes of the eye lens, leading to the formation of cataracts. Much of this free-radical damage may be preventable by nutritional supplementation, the wearing of protective eyeglasses and electromagnetic rebalancing (see "Step 2: Rebalance Electromagnetics").

Dietary changes can be helpful as well. Free radicals in water can be avoided by not drinking chlorinated and fluoridated water or waters polluted by industry and agriculture. Heat processed oils, contain free radicals; cold-pressed oils, like extra virgin olive oil, do not.

Eating a diet rich in all antioxidants, carotenes and Vitamin A can lower the incidence of cataracts, according to a study published in the *British Medical Journal* (see "Step 6: Remove Heavy Metals or Other Toxins from the Body," for further information).

It has been reported that the greatest single cause of cataracts is linked to the body's inability to cope with sugar. Lactose (milk sugar) is the worst offender identified, followed closely by refined white sugar. Other studies have linked cataract formation to consumption of milk products, smoking and deficiencies in enzymes important in digestion, which convert food into nutritional forms usable by the body.

Total Eyebright-C™ contains many of the nutrients that support lens and eye health.

MACULA

For people over 55 years old, macular degeneration is the leading cause of severe vision loss in both the U.S. and Europe. Macular degeneration is the third-leading cause of loss of vision among those over 65.

Macular degeneration is a condition where the macula, the central area of the retina, deteriorates, resulting in a loss of sharp vision. Loss of vision is accompanied by leaking or hemorrhaging of fluid from tiny blood vessel networks that develop under the center of the retina. This condition results in scarring and eventual loss of vision.

Macular degeneration is believed to be caused by free-radical damage similar to the damage that induces cataracts. Structural factors that can affect poor vision include temporal bone pressure on the nerves to the eyes, neck tension and pressure on occipital lobes of the brain interfering with messages getting to visual centers, for which craniosacral and chiropractic therapies have been shown to be very helpful.

Loss of vision usually occurs slowly and progresses slowly, but may occurs suddenly. Color and peripheral vision aren't affected. Bad dietary habits can deplete nutrients essential to eye health and promote excessive free-radical damage to the eyes.

You can improve or slow the progression of macular degeneration by avoiding alcohol (with the possible exception of moderate wine consumption), cigarette smoke, fats and oils that are heat-processed (choose cold-pressed or expeller-expressed oils), fried foods, hamburgers, luncheon meats, roasted nuts and all refined sugars.

Choose organic, unrefined, whole foods, especially legumes, yellow-orange vegetables, spinach and amaranth. Cold-pressed, extra-virgin olive oil can multiply your intake of lutein from spinach fourfold. Eat plenty of raw fruits and vegetables rich in Vitamins E and C. You must also add flavonoid-rich blueberries, blackberries and cherries to your diet.

Total Eyebright-M™ contains many of the nutrients that support the macula and eye health.

IMMUNE SYSTEM:
PROTECTIVE NUTRIENTS AND PHYTOCHEMICALS

The oxidizing agents called free radicals react to healthy cells and tissues, potentially causing damage. Free radicals have been linked to over 60 degenerative diseases. Sources of free radicals include cellular respiration, pollutant chemicals from food, water and air, sun exposure, x-rays, heavy metals such as mercury, cadmium and lead, cigarette smoke and alcohol.

Reducing exposure and increasing intake of protective antioxidant nutrients and phytochemicals can lower the risks of free-radical-caused health problems by protecting against the formation of free radicals, protecting the cells against the damage of oxidative chemicals and enhancing the immune system.

Phytochemicals aren't yet classified as substances essential for sustaining life, but they have been identified as containing properties for aiding in disease prevention.

Phytochemicals are associated with the prevention of at least four of the leading causes of death in the United States: cardiovascular disease, hypertension, diabetes and cancer. Phytochemicals are involved in many actions that help prevent cell damage, decrease cholesterol levels and inhibit disease processes. Protective phytochemicals are found abundantly in legumes, herbs, fruits and vegetables. Legume, fruit and vegetable consumption in population studies have been consistently shown to reduce the risk of many diseases.

The FDA won't allow claims that supplements help prevent cancer, even though the National Cancer Institute is telling us to eat foods containing these same substances for the same purpose – to prevent cancer. We don't make this claim. We simply show what various nutrients do. The FDA is on record as saying that "supplements are disincentives to drug development." You can't patent what nature makes. You can only patent what humans invent, and patents are where the big money is.

We formulated a synergistic blend of nutrients called Total Protect™ (veg), which contains many of the supportive phytonutrients and nutrients for the immune system.

We also formulated a product containing 23 nutrients and phytonutrients (emphasizing sprouts and whole foods) that help alkalize the body, called Total Veggie™ (veg). This is the nutrient blend that gives you all of your vegetables in a pill form. There is no longer any excuse why you can't get the protective vegetables the American Cancer Society recommends.

STOMACH

A strong stomach isn't only essential for good digestion, but is essential to defend the body against invading viruses, bacteria and other unfriendly organisms. A strong stomach will defend the body against incompletely digested food particles that could enter the bloodstream and weaken other systems and organs or trigger over-reactions in the immune system.

We formulated and use a product called Total Upper GI™ that contains the nutrients to help prevent the symptoms of a hiatal hernia and GERD (gastroesophageal reflex disease.)

KIDNEYS

The kidneys are responsible for disposing of wastes from the body. They filter blood and return water and other purified substances back into the blood. The excretion product of the kidneys is urine, which is stored in the bladder until it's released from the body.

Kidney stones are caused by precipitates of mineral salts from the urine. 70% of kidney stones are composed of calcium oxalate and are caused by inadequate water intake or excesses in consumption of coffee, soft drinks and high oxalate foods such as spinach.

As our kidneys age, they don't excrete phosphorus as well. Because meat is high in phosphorus, our meat consumption should decline and leafy vegetable consumption should increase after age 40.

The kidneys must be functioning properly to effectively eliminate waste products and toxins from the body. Drink at least eight glasses of water a day and get adequate exercise to keep your kidneys functioning well.

MALE HEALTH

Nearly 30 million men in the U.S. suffer occasional to chronic impotence. Although most are over 40, younger men also can have problems. By age 60, one-third of all men are affected.

Over 85% of all cases are believed to have physical causes. Anxiety, impaired blood flow to erectile tissue, impaired nerve functions, hormone imbalance, high blood pressure, diabetes, vasectomy, alcohol, smoking and many medications can interfere with potency. The most common drugs that can produce impotence are antidepressants, antihistamines, antihypertensives, diuretics, narcotics, sedatives, stomach acid inhibitors and ulcer medications. A diet high in animal fats, carbohydrates and refined sugar, age-related decline in digestive health and malabsorption of nutrients are believed to be primary causes of declines in male health. Alcohol intake impairs the body's production of testosterone and may cause the male hormonal equivalent of menopause.

Total Male™ (veg) is a synergistic formula for male health that we formulated and use in our practices. Maca (Lepidum Meyenii), called the Andean Ginseng, is one of its ingredients used for its invigorating properties. Maca's lysine and arginine can help promote fertility and sexual desire. Maca's sterols, brassycosterol, ergosterol, carnpesterol, delta 7.22 ergostadienol and especially sitosterol and glucosinolates can help balance reproductive hormones.

PROSTATE

The prostate secretes an alkaline prostate fluid that forms the largest part of the semen. Benign prostatic hypertrophy (BPH) affects 10 million men, half over the age of 50, and 75% over the age of 70. BPH is mainly attributed to hormone changes associated with aging, the decline of testosterone production and the increase of estradiol and prolactin. This imbalance creates an increase of dihydrotestosterone within the prostate, which promotes prostate enlargement.

We have formulated and use several products to give proper nutrition for male health. Zinc is also very important for proper prostate function and protection.

FEMALE HEALTH

The uterus in a non-pregnant woman is a pear-shaped organ joining the vagina at the cervix. It's composed of smooth muscle and mucous membrane lining. It undergoes periodic development and degeneration with the menstrual cycle.

30%—50% of all women suffer pain or discomfort during menstruation. Menstrual cramps (dysmenorrhea) were once thought of as a minor complaint that was "all in a woman's head." Present thinking suggests that cramping is caused by excess production of hormone-like prostaglandins following declines in progesterone levels.

10% of women afflicted with dysmenorrhea have symptoms severe enough that they cannot perform normal activities. Sharp, viselike pains stem from tightening of uterine muscle, poor blood circulation and impaired oxygenation of uterine muscle. Excess estrogen worsens these problems because estrogen increases salt and fluid retention.

Unbalanced estrogen-progesterone levels associated with menstruation can cause headaches, irritability, mood swings, depression, weight gain from excess water retention and loss of sex drive.

Many women in Asia, Yucatan and Mexico are fortunate enough to go through menopause with few problems. Other cultures aren't so fortunate. The symptoms of perimenopause and menopause can exaggerate PMS problems, along with irregular menstrual cycles, more irritability, anxiety, depression, bloating, food cravings and breast tenderness. Menopausal symptoms are caused by erratic estrogen dominance as the body's supply of progesterone declines.

• •

About Menopause

Symptoms include memory loss, irritability, depression, water retention, and weight gain. Vaginal walls become drier and thinner, and sexual interest may decline. This is accompanied by increased susceptibility to yeast and bacterial infections, fibrocystic breasts, breast cancer, fibroids, or endometrial cancer. Sugar, alcohol, smoking, coffee and tea consumption can worsen symptoms.

• •

Becoming informed about helpful lifestyle changes, adopting a natural whole foods diet, taking nutritional supplements and regular exercise can help maintain female health.

ESTROGEN DOMINANCE

The female organs produce estrogen and progesterone in what sometimes seems to be a tug of war during a woman's cycle, as concentrations of each hormone fluctuate. Since estrogen prevails for most of the cycle, it creates a condition commonly referred to as estrogen dominance. This imbalance happens both in PMS and in menopause, when estrogen replacement therapy (ERT) is given.

Symptoms of estrogen dominance include: water retention, breast swelling, fibrocystic breasts, pre-menstrual mood swings and depression, loss of sex drive, heavy or irregular periods, uterine fibroids, craving for sweets and fat deposition in the hips and thighs. Progesterone is an important hormone that balances estrogen.

THE GOOD NEWS ABOUT NATURAL SUPPORT

A growing number of doctors believe that if natural products were used, medical risks and side effects would be considerably lessened. Research using hormones from natural sources have the benefits of synthetics but fewer side effects. A significant finding showed that natural progesterone eliminated the adverse effects of the synthetic progestins on blood-fats and cholesterol levels.

PHYTOESTROGENS

Plant phytoestrogens don't carry the risks of estrogen replacement therapy, yet have the ability to exert a weak estrogenic activity when they bind to estrogen receptors. Phytoestrogens are found in some 300 foods and in some herbs including: flaxseeds, tofu, cabbage, alfalfa, fennel, dong quai, red raspberry, black cohosh, chaste-tree berries (vitex), red clover, wild yam and licorice root. Since the plant hormones have weak estrogenic activity, they're able to eliminate some of the symptoms of menopause and decrease the risk for osteoporosis. Used together synergistically, they're even more powerful.

If plant estrogens provide weak activity where there was none before, does that increase the risk for breast cancer? There is no conclusive evidence that they do. That could be due to the natural quality of the estrogen, and also that plant estrogens may be exerting other beneficial effects. For instance, these plant estrogens bind to an enzyme called estrogen synthetase, thus inhibiting production of the estrogen in the body and potentially offering additional protection in this manner.

NATURAL SUPPORT FOR OSTEOPOROSIS

One of the reasons the trial on Hormone Replacement Therapy (HRT) wasn't halted earlier was because hip fractures decreased with estrogen. Both phytoestrogens and natural progesterone can support healthy bones. The bioactivity of several phytoestrogens in preventing bone loss has been demonstrated in a well-recognized model of postmenopausal bone loss. Researchers note that osteoporosis has been reversed in women as much as 16 years past menopause, using natural progesterone in combination with other dietary factors, and exercise.

Phytoestrogens, proper calcium/magnesium intake and natural progesterone cream can offer a lot in the way of support for both pre- and postmenopausal women. Studies of over 16,000 women have discredited the notion that synthetic hormone replacement therapy is the best option for menopausal women. The natural alternatives certainly don't carry the risks that accompany the medical hormone replacement, an increasing number of women these days want a healthier alternative.

We formulated and use a synergistic blend of nutrients called Total Fem™ (veg) to support female health.

SEX DRIVE

Overall health and energy can influence sexual behavior and sexual drive. Sexual vitality can also influence overall health, including benefiting the immune system. High blood pressure, atherosclerosis, peripheral vascular disease, diabetes, hyperthyroidism, hypothyroidism, low hormone levels and psychological issues can affect potency. Fears of intimacy, fears of sexual intercourse, performance anxieties, depression, low self-esteem, guilt, repressed anger, boredom and anxiety can also be factors. Common drugs may cause impotence, including alcohol, nicotine, antihistamines, antidepressants, antihypertensives, diuretics, narcotics, ulcer medications and stomach acid inhibitors.

Both men and women are subject to sexual dysfunction. It's simply a matter of circulation. Low testosterone levels in women also affect sexual drive in the same way a man's sex drive is impaired by testosterone levels.

Poor diet and malabsorption of nutrients are believed to be primary causes of declines in male and female health. Total Arginine™ is a synergistic formula for male and female health, containing many of these vital nutrients for circulation enhancement.

BONES

Osteoporosis is a major, disabling epidemic affecting an estimated 20 million Americans. The United States has a yearly rate of over one million fractures caused by osteoporosis – the highest rate of osteoporotic fractures in the world.

The standard American diet, which contains food grown on depleted soils, has left Americans deficient in nutrients crucial for bone health. Compounding the problem, the standard American diet consists of high sodium, protein, sugar and processed foods, which causes further calcium loss. This diet has an acidifying effect on metabolism, drawing calcium out of bone tissue to buffer this overly acidic condition.

Bone is more than just a collection of inert calcium crystals. It's an active, living tissue, constantly remodeling and rebuilding itself in a flux of biochemical change. Since bone is an active living tissue, it has a direct and constant need for a wide range of nutritional support. Bone health is dependent on a large combination of nutrients, including Vitamins B6, C, D, K, folic acid, as well as the minerals magnesium, manganese, boron, zinc, copper, strontium, and silicon and natural sources of progesterone.

A deficiency of several different nutrients can lead to osteoporosis or other calcium deficient conditions. A good approach to building strong and healthy bones would include a calcium formula, blended with all known synergistic factors helpful in promoting bone health, to your diet. Exercise should be moderate for those with osteoporosis.

Our formulation, Total Calcium™ (veg), contains many of the nutrients to support healthy bones.

JOINTS

Rheumatoid Arthritis (RA) affects over two million people in the United States, usually between the ages of 20-50, though 200,000 children in the U.S. are also affected. Symptoms of RA include: night sweats, depression, fatigue, low grade fever, weakness, joint stiffness and painfully swollen joints.

15% of the total U.S. population is affected with some form of arthritis, according to the National Institute of Health. One-third of all adults in the United States show evidence of osteoarthritis in the hand, knee or hip. By age 75, 3/4 of all adults have signs of the disease.

Osteoarthritis is a degenerative condition of the larger weight-bearing joints associated with bony growths, soft cysts on bones and joints and cartilage deterioration. Symptoms include: mild early morning stiffness, stiffness after resting, pain that worsens after joint use, restricted joint function, tenderness, swelling and creaking and cracking of joints.

Arthritis may be caused by many factors, including stress, joint instability, hormonal changes, environmental and psychological factors, aging, excess weight, general wear and tear, inadequate diet and exercise, food sensitivities and allergies, high animal fat diets, leaky gut, abnormal bowel function and many infections (including *Candida albicans*).

Natural approaches to preventing and improving arthritis emphasize proper diet and nutrition, exercise, nutritional supplements, weight reduction and identification of food allergies and sensitivities. Proper diets are rich in fresh fruits and vegetables, cold water fish, nuts and whole grains (with the exception of wheat). Arthritis sufferers must also cut down or eliminate hydrogenated fats, processed foods, non-organic foods, fatty meats, eggs, dairy products, caffeine, tobacco, alcohol and sugars.

● ●

Avoid Nightshade Plants to Ease Arthritis Pain
A survey of persons avoiding the nightshade plants alone showed that 44% had a positive response and 28% had a "marked positive response." The nightshade plants to avoid are tomatoes, tobacco, white potatoes, all peppers (except black pepper), eggplant, etc.

● ●

Natural approaches to easing arthritis pain include supplementing with nutritional factors that have antioxidant and safe anti-inflammatory results. Natural approaches avoid the side effects of drugs and also include nutrition that helps protect, build and repair healthy bones, joints and synovial fluid and helps build and repair permeability of the intestinal wall.

Nutritional supplements discussed below are natural and safe ways for you to protect cartilage, repair damage and rebuild healthy bones, cartilage, tendons, ligaments and joint fluid.

Special herbs and nutrients help reduce inflammation and pain associated with arthritic problems and allergies. Drugs, taken for inflammatory pain, relieve symptoms but cause side-effects that can damage the gut lining, causing leaky gut, as well as destroy the cartilage lining of joints.

Our formulation, Total Inflam™ (veg), contains many of the nutrients for support of inflammation and reduction of pain.

MANGANESE DEFICIENCY

Current farming practices, soil erosion, soil leaching and soil exhaustion all contribute to depleting the amount of manganese available to leafy green vegetables and whole grains, our normal sources of this trace mineral. Processing further depletes our intake of this essential mineral.

Corn germ can contain as much as 10 mg per 100 gm, but corn flakes contain only 0.04 mg. Other dramatic losses occur in the processing of wheat.

Hair analysis has suggested that manganese deficiency, which is common among older men, has been implicated in atherosclerosis and is suspected of being a cause of diabetes. Manganese deficiency impairs sugar metabolism and lowers glucose tolerance.

A manganese deficiency may also lead to confusion, convulsions, eye problems, hearing problems, heart disorders, hypertension, memory loss, dizziness, pancreatic damage, profuse perspiration, rapid pulse, tooth grinding, breast ailments and osteoporosis. Many of these symptoms may be caused by heavy metal intoxication. Manganese and Vitamin B6 help block and release metal poisoning behind these symptoms.

Manganese is essential for healthy skin, bone, cartilage formation, lubricating synovial fluid in joints, glucose tolerance, activating superoxide dismutase (SOD), protein and fat metabolism, healthy nerves, healthy brain function, muscular strength, a healthy immune system and normal reproduction.

Manganese can help reduce fatigue, aid muscle reflexes, prevent osteoporosis, improve memory, help those with recurrent dizziness and reduce nervous irritability.

Supplementation helps activate enzymes for the body's use of Biotin, Vitamin B1 and Vitamin C, and is important in the thyroid's production of thyroxin. It's also necessary for proper digestion and utilization of food.

MOTHER NATURE'S ANSWER

CMO (Cetyl myristoleate) may be nature's answer to arthritis, multiple sclerosis, fibromyalgia and lupus because of its ability to normalize an overactive immune system.

In 1971, the researcher H.W. Diehl made a startling discovery: Swiss Albino mice carried natural CMO, which prevented them from getting arthritis! Diehl then demonstrated that CMO also prevented arthritis in experimental animals susceptible to arthritis.

Failing to interest pharmaceutical companies in his discovery, Diehl tried CMO on his own arthritis to find that 20 days later, his arthritic symptoms were dramatically alleviated, along with remission in headaches and bronchitis.

His daughter, hundreds of friends and members of his congregation began taking CMO and reported improvements in rheumatoid arthritis, lower-back pain, tendinitis, bursitis, fibromyalgia, carpal tunnel syndrome, milder forms of joint and soft tissue inflammation and many other conditions. In Siemandi's placebo-controlled trial of 431 patients, over half of the patients taking CMO showed 75% improvement. Other clinical work has shown even greater results with the addition of liver detoxification, enzyme therapy and natural anti-inflammatories – raising CMO's success rate from 58% to nearly 80%.

CMO appears to normalize the immune system and stop the body's attack on its own healthy tissues. It seems not to matter what the autoimmune attack trigger is, whether it's a food allergy, excessive fat, or foreign substances from microbes. CMO also seems to have a lubricating effect, allowing stiff joints to move more easily. Therefore, we formulated a synergistic blend referred to as Total CMO™.

120

MITOCHONDRIA, OUR CELL'S ENERGY FURNACE

Next to pain, fatigue is the most common patient complaint. About 90 million people worldwide, and 3 million Americans, are afflicted by Chronic Fatigue Syndrome (CFS/CFIDS). Fibromyalgia (FM) leaves another 3 to 6 million people with chronic tiredness and pain. The National Academy of Medicine estimates that 15% of the U.S. population suffers from fatigue associated with chemical sensitivities, sometimes called "Multiple Chemical Sensitivities."
Other causes include nutritional deficiencies, overwork, multiple infections, lowered immune function, mitochondria injury, aging, vaccinations, abnormal muscle tension, heavy metals and drug, tobacco or alcohol abuse.

The mitochondria are the energy furnaces of the body. When the mitochondria make insufficient adenosine triphosphate (ATP) – our energy fuel – we have inadequate energy for our bodies.

In CFS, most energy production is believed to be diverted to support immune function, with little left over for other needs. This leads to premature aging, muscle wasting, fatigue, sleep disturbances, mental dysfunction, pain and other problems.

Shortly after exercise begins, CFS/CFIDS people reach the anaerobic threshold known as, "hitting the wall," the wall that marathon runners experience after prolonged physical exertion.
People with CFS are tired before they run the race. They may live close to the anaerobic threshold due to "metabolic injury" involving the mitochondria, where excessive lactic acid is associated with pain and fatigue.

When we supplement with nutrients that support healthy functioning of the mitochondria, we find that energy production is maximized, creating energy for more satisfying and active lives. Total Mitochondria™ (veg) contains the best combination of these nutrients, needed for mitochondria and energy support, we have ever seen.

FROM THE MOMENT WE'RE BORN, WE'RE GETTING OLD

Aging is partly caused by the deterioration of our cells' abilities to reproduce. Cells die and replace themselves, in normal and youthful ways, at least every two years of cellular life.

Eventually, however, our millions of cells begin to deteriorate and grow old, and we grow old with them. Cells can be rejuvenated, if provided with proper nourishment through nutritional support.

Aging is accompanied by decreases in Growth Hormone (GH) levels. After our teenage years, GH levels decline at about 14% per decade. By 50 years of age, it's believed that GH production may virtually stop. Cell replacement, tissue repair, healing, organ health, bone strength, brain function, enzyme production and the health of hair, nails and skin all require adequate amounts of GH. By supplementing your diet with the amino acids and vitamins that stimulate the release of growth hormone, production can be brought back to the levels of a young adult.

Growth hormone plays a key role in the youthful body's growth and repair processes. It enhances protein synthesis for muscle growth, helps burn fat, improves resistance to disease and accelerates wound healing, among other functions.

GH replacement therapy has reported these benefits:
- A general enhancement of health
- More positive outlooks
- Decreased body fat
- A rebuilding of muscle mass
- Increased ability to exercise
- Increased energy levels
- Improved memory and mental alertness
- Improved skin appearance and texture
- New hair growth and color restoration in some individuals
- Improved lung function
- Increased bone mass in osteoporosis
- Strengthening of the immune system
- Enhanced sex drive

Since insulin suppresses GH release and the greatest release is in the first hour-and-a-half of sleep, it's important not to eat sugar in any form close to bedtime. It's also important to restrict sugar intake during the day and not to eat before exercising so you won't interfere with growth hormone release.

The father of the free-radical theory of aging, Denham Harman, theorized that the degenerative disorders we normally associate with aging aren't inevitable with just the passage of time. Instead, much of the damage caused by excess free radicals can be prevented by the use of supplemental and dietary anti oxidants.

SUMMARY

- Poor diet, which leads to poor digestion and interferes with the body's ability to nourish itself, can be repaired.
- Nourishing foods grown on rich soils, not the depleted and polluted soils of conventional foods, will replenish your body.
- Junk foods, processed foods, anything canned, soft drinks and sugar are close to nutritional voids (depleted of minerals and nutrients and polluted with chemical additives and pesticide residues).
- Hearts and arteries, weakened by improper diet and lifestyle, can be replenished. Losses in vision, from diet and pollution, can be corrected. Once the whole body and the whole system are replenished, the body has all it chemically needs, to rebuild and repair itself.
- Proper nutritional support with synergistic nutrition is a must for almost all people to get adequate levels of nutrients at this time.

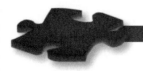

Step 3C
Reduce Infective Organisms in the Body

We're going to look at organisms that cause infection a little differently from how you may have considered them in the past. Traditional western medicine has practiced name-and-blame in their approach to health care. It's actually been, "disease-care" more than healthcare.

Chiropractors and naturopaths have concentrated on building up the "host" (you) more than treating your symptoms or infective process. They teach that the body has an innate intelligence that, if not interfered with, will actually seek health and wellness.

What we've found in our research and practice is that there are six major stressors that weaken us and allow the manifestation of disease. One of those is the load of infective organisms in the body. You may think that it's an either-or situation: either you have a virus or a yeast infection or you don't. They're either in your body and you're sick, or they're not in your body and you're fine.

The fact is, there are said to be over 500 good types of bacteria living in our intestines. These bacteria are very important to our health, and when they're killed off with antibiotics, we can develop diarrhea, constipation, etc.

Viruses, bacteria, yeast, parasites and more can all be inside you without manifesting symptoms you recognize as disease. Their presence can, in fact, cause a constant stress and manifest any number of symptoms and diseases over time.

Our philosophy is to build you up with the *6 Steps To Wellness* and not wait until a disease manifests itself or even until you show symptoms.

We use multiple forms of testing to identify proper, optimal health treatment and to prevent disease in the body. Among these are muscle response testing, darkfield evaluation (live blood analysis), blood tests, urine, saliva, electrodermal testing and hair analysis.

In our offices, utilizing all 6 Steps helps build the immune system and help the body function optimally. In this section, we'll examine different possible infective organisms and point out specific nutrition that has proven effective.

WHEN THE YEAST RISES

Candida albicans is a natural inhabitant of the mouth, throat, genital tract, vagina and skin. In healthy people, the population of candida is small and kept in balance by a strong, well-functioning immune system and by the presence of competing, friendly bacteria such as bifido and acidophilus. Many conditions cause this fungal yeast to multiply, and overgrowth causes symptoms often confused with other diseases.

According to C. Orian Truss, MD, in <u>The Missing Diagnosis</u>, candida has been known to produce symptoms that mimic virtually every known disease condition. Hiatal hernia, which forces the stomach into the esophagus, and a malfunctioning ileocecal valve, which allows backward movement of the bowel, also have reputations for being "great mimickers."

• • • • • • • • • • • • • • • • • • •

Common Symptoms of Yeast Infection:
- Constipation
- Diarrhea
- Colitis
- Stomach pain
- Headache
- Bad breath
- Rectal itching
- Mood swings
- Memory loss
- Prostatitis
- Canker sores
- Heartburn
- Muscle-joint pain

- Sore throat
- Congestion
- Coughing
- Clogged sinuses
- Numbness in the face, arms or legs
- Tingling sensations
- Night sweats
- Acne
- Severe itching
- PMS
- Burning tongue
- White spots on the tongue and mouth
- Chronic fatigue
- Vaginitis
- Kidney and bladder infections
- Arthritis
- Depression
- Hyperactivity
- Hypothyroidism
- Diabetes
- Athlete's foot
- Jock itch
- Intolerance of contact with rubber, petroleum products, tobacco, exhaust fumes and chemical odors
- Adrenal problems

Symptoms may worsen in damp and moldy environments and after eating foods containing sugar and yeast.

John Ely, PhD, reported that mercury accumulation results in one important cause of overgrowth that doesn't respond to most treatment.

We've long noticed that the toxic processes of fungal yeasts appear to feed off heavy metals and tend to improve with decrease in metal overloads. Heavy metals and infective organisms pair up. (See Step 6: *Remove Heavy Metals or Other Toxins from the Body.*)

Other causes of fungal overgrowth can be found from the use of: cortisone which is prescribed for skin conditions such as eczema and psoriasis. Additionally, repeated use of antibiotics, ulcer medications and oral contraceptives also may cause fungal overgrowth. Conditions such as pregnancy, cancer, poor dietary habits, including eating foods with pesticide residues and preservatives, margarine with hydrogenated fats, alcohol use, chemotherapy, and radiation, also injure or destroy T-cells and can increase yeast overgrowth.

As fungal yeast overgrows, the B-complex declines, especially biotin, synthesized by friendly bacteria like acidophilus. Biotin synthesis by acidophilus is linked to controlled and normal growth of unfriendly bacteria. In overgrowth conditions, yeast changes into mycelial forms that penetrate intestinal tissues with threadlike arms. Waste products, such as alcohol, acetaldehyde and vinegar, enter the bloodstream, resulting in food sensitivities and allergic and toxic reactions. Other toxic debris and undigested foods can enter the bloodstream, causing further allergies.

• •

To Combat Yeast Overgrowth, Avoid:
- Sugars, in all forms
- Sucrose
- Dextrose
- Fructose
- Fruit juices
- Lactose in milk products
- Potatoes
- Honey
- Maple syrup
- Molasses
- Most fruit, except berries
- Fresh pineapple
- Papaya
- Grain-based products
- Breads
- Baked goods

• •

People with yeast overgrowth usually become sensitive to fermented foods such as vinegar and foods containing cheeses, grapes and mushrooms.

Conventional meats, dairy and poultry products can foster yeast overgrowth because of antibiotic residues. 50% of all antibiotics used in America are fed to our livestock to increase weight gain by keeping down infection.

Specific nutritional support is given for any stress area where a fungal yeast or bacterial infection is indicated by testing. Our formulation that we use is Total Yeast Redux™ (veg): Nutritional Support for Fungal-Yeast and Bacteria.

• • • • • • • • • • • • • • • • • • • •

A Case of Fungal Yeast Infection and Fibromyalgia

I'm a 55-year-old woman who for the last eight years has felt like an 80-year-old woman lots of days. I got diagnosed with fibromyalgia at the Mayo Clinic in 1991. They basically told me to live with the pain, as they do not know what causes it, and there is nothing to treat it with. I've been to many doctors, about 15 in all. Not until I heard Dr. Brimhall's lectures did I know that I finally found doctors I wanted to treat me. I was to the point of being desperate and depressed and told my husband to take me to Superstition Mountains so I could jump off because I could not stand the pain. I started seeing the Brimhall Clinic on March 25, 1998. I have never seen such caring and compassionate doctors. I just want to thank the doctors and all of their staff (and the wonderful free hugs) for helping me get on the road to good health and giving me a feeling "THERE IS HELP OUT THERE." I have a clearer head when I wake up in the morning. I don't feel bloated anymore and hardly have any diarrhea. I have more energy during the day. I just wish I had found Brimhall's Wellness Center sooner.

—LaVonne S.

● ○ ○ ● ○ ● ● ● ● ● ● ● ● ● ● ● ● ● ● ● ●

IT MUST BE A VIRUS

Virus infections play roles in such harmful conditions as heart disease, AIDS, bladder infections, bronchitis, chickenpox, cold sores, the common cold, croup, diarrhea, ear infection, eye infections, German measles, hepatitis, herpes virus conditions, flu, measles, meningitis, mononucleosis, mumps, pancreatitis, pneumonia, Reye's Syndrome, shingles, tonsillitis and warts.

Many factors play roles in encouraging infections, including alternating-current (AC) electromagnetic fields, diet, stress, overwork, fatigue, and thermal shock in climate change.

The enemy is widespread. Let's look at some of the most prevalent viruses.

Forty to 80% of the U.S. population has been estimated to be infected by herpes simplex (HSV-1), either showing as cold sores or with silent infection showing no symptoms. Once the herpes viruses enter the body, they become permanent residents, frequently hiding in the nerves, although they rarely present as problems after the age of 50. More than 90 viruses belong to this family.

Varicella-zoster causes chickenpox and shingles. Epstein-Barr virus (EBV) causes mononucleosis and is found in people with Chronic Fatigue Syndrome. Cytomegalovirus (CMV) can be carried without symptoms, but can have terrible effects on people with compromised immune systems and infants. HSV-1 causes cold sores, skin eruptions, and eventually presents as varicella-zoster or another form causing shingles. If HSV-1 infects the eye, it can cause scarring and loss of vision.

Herpes simplex II (HSV-2) is a common sexually transmitted virus that can be silent (no symptoms or effect) or result in inflammation of the liver. This virus is the cause of genital herpes in women, which can show as blisters on the clitoris, rectum, cervix or vagina. This family of viruses is known to lie dormant, sometimes erupting once a year or even less frequently, triggered sometimes by other illnesses, sun exposure, fatigue, stress or other factors.

Chronic Fatigue Syndrome (CFS) has been linked with EBV. It normally reduces daily activity by at least 50% for at least a period of six months and has such symptoms as aching muscles and joints, anxiety, depression, difficulties in concentration, irritability, muscle spasms and disabling fatigue.

However, Chronic Fatigue Syndrome may be problematic because, like CMV, it's known to be a problem in immune-compromised individuals. The immune system may be so weak that the virus takes its toll on the rest of the body.

More than 200 viruses can cause the common cold and flu, which can lead to bronchitis and pneumonia. In people over 60, flu infections are the fifth-leading cause of death. H. influenza type B virus, poliovirus, rubella (measles virus), and bacteria such as streptococcus pneumonia and type B streptococcus, as well as fungal yeasts, are all causes of meningitis, which affects the meninges between the brain and skull.

Cocksaxie virus, also associated with CFS, has been implicated in heart disease under nutritionally deficient circumstances, where it has been described as attacking heart muscle and causing heart failure. In our clinical practice, we've found many of our patients with heart problems also have had viral infections. We believe that heart viruses can weaken the heart in just days and destroy a heart in only 90 days.

• •

A Case of Chronic Fatigue and Virus

When I first came in, I had two known viruses, Epstein-Barr and Parvo. These caused severe fatigue, so severe that I could not stand for five minutes without needing to sit. My muscles and joints were in constant pain. I had insomnia, weight gain, nausea, shaking of my body, fever and depression. The first thing I noticed when I started was how helpful everyone at the Brimhall Wellness Center was. They really do care for your comfort and health. As my progress continued, I would have my ups and downs, which is very normal in the healing process. I was so jazzed to finally be able to exercise after not being able to for three years. I can truly say that all the methods used have helped me greatly, and I feel 90% better than I did in only three-and-a-half months! Thank you, Dr. Brimhall and staff, for all you have done for me! You guys are the greatest! You are a Godsend to me!

—Lori Anne M.

A variety of diagnostic tools can be used to identify organs and body systems that may be under stress from viral infections: kinesiology can ask the body where stress patterns are located, and the cold laser and Frequency Modulator can be used as diagnostic and treatment tools. Your symptoms can reveal a lot. Although we're not symptom-chasers, we listen to the clues they leave.

Specific nutritional support is given for any stress area where a viral infection is suspected as indicated by testing. Total Virx™ (veg) contains many of the nutrients to help support the body in viral infections.

YOU PARASITE!

We're exposed to a variety of organisms with the potential to drain life energy from our bodies. Parasites are one of the biggest factors in lowering our immune system's ability to protect us. They weaken us and hinder our defenses. These organisms deplete the body's stores of nutrients as well. It's wise to supplement with the vital vitamins, minerals and the nutrients we need. It's also essential to have a strong and healthy immune system.

A Case of Parasites and Heavy Metal

Laura was referred in March 2002 by her brother, Juan. We were told she had a skin condition, was very tired and depressed. Upon meeting Laura, she seemed reserved and unable to communicate well, although we were told she spoke English fluently. Laura had a rash that appeared like a burn all over her face, hands and chest for over 10 years. Laura's brother said she had spent a lot of time in her bedroom over the last 10 years because she didn't want people to see her. Recently, she had missed a lot of work. Laura tested positive for parasites and lead. Giving Laura a magnet to help balance her electromagnetic problem we found and DSF™ quickly began to restore her energy along with the following Brimhall formulations: Homocysteine Redux™, Total Enzymes™, Total Leaky Gut™, Total Para™, Total Probiotics™, Total Lead™, and Black Current Seed Oil. By June, Laura had shown significant improvement and began to wear makeup for the first time. Laura evolved into a beautiful woman with a bubbly personality and has recently married. Her rash has cleared up completely.

— Colin R. D., DC

DO YOU HAVE PARASITES?

Conservative estimates suggest that 10% of the U.S. population is infected with parasites. However, a John Hopkins study of random samples from blood tests found that 18% of all blood samples showed parasite infections.

Roundworm parasites infect 25% of the world's population. In the U.S., roundworms are prevalent in the Appalachian and nearby areas.

Worldwide, 30% of all people show evidence of Giardia lamblia infection, a highly contagious parasite transmitted by fecal contamination, contacted by drinking or swimming in contaminated surface waters in lakes and streams, and by contact with wildlife, cats and dogs.

In Kansas, the contamination of groundwater has been reported to be 86%. In Arizona, 50% of Native Americans living on reservations have parasite infections.

Half of all people diagnosed with irritable bowel syndrome have been found to have intestinal parasites. When treated for parasites, the majority of people with irritable bowel saw their symptoms disappear.

Of those diagnosed with Chronic Fatigue Syndrome, 82% of those treated for parasites were relieved of their symptoms. In patients with CFS, 33% showed evidence of Giardia infection.

Parasites can be silent in the body or cause a wide variety of symptoms that mimic other diseases. Many unrecognized causes of ill health have been attributed to parasite infections.

• • • • • • • • • • • • • • • • • • • •

How to Avoid Parasites

Pets

- De-worm pets regularly
- Keep your pets and their sleeping areas clean
- Don't let pets lick your face (a neat trick)
- Don't let pets lick your dishes
- Don't walk barefoot near your pets
- Don't sleep with or near your pets
- Wash your hands after petting your animals

Washing and Food

- Wash your hands after gardening and using the bathroom

- Wash utensils well after cutting meat and fish
- Wash your hands after handling meat and fish
- Wash vegetables thoroughly and soak them in fresh water with a few drops of citrus seed extract
- Use wooden cutting boards (many microbes can't live on wood)
- Use separate cutting boards for meats/fish and other foods
- Don't eat raw fish (as in sushi) or raw meat

Travel

- Take protective herbs
- Be cautious with local foods in underdeveloped countries (infected immigrant workers who handle food and the popularity of ethnic raw foods such as sushi, sashimi and ceviche contribute to higher risks of parasites)

We have also used the Frequency Modulator's and cold laser's special frequencies to help reduce parasites.

Total Para™ (Veg) is a special nutrient support formulated to help reduce Parasites.

A CASE FOR THE DEFENSE

Your first line of defense is a healthy energy field and a strong immune system. The thymus, parotid, lymph nodes, spleen, bone marrow and tonsils all play essential roles. Specialized white blood cells, lymphocytes, phagocytes, killer T-cells, antibodies, interferon, and lactoferrin also play major roles in immune function.

Your skin acts as a first barrier against unfriendly invasions.

The immune system provides a secondary defense against attacking microorganisms. Mucus secretions, including tears, gastric acid secretions and saliva from the parotid gland, are part of this defense.

Dietary habits can damage immune system function. All forms of refined sugar interfere with the white blood cells' ability to destroy unfriendly bacteria. Alcohol weakens a wide variety of immune responses, and excessive dietary fat lowers natural killer T-cell activity.

Phytochemicals are associated with the prevention or treatment of at least four of the leading causes of death in the United States: diabetes, cancer, cardiovascular disease and hypertension. These protective substances are found abundantly in fruits and vegetables.

Total Multimune™: Nutrients is a supplement designed to support the immune system.

• • • • • • • • • • • • • • • • • • • •

A Case of Fatigue

I was sleeping 10 hours a night, but feeling so fatigued I had to sleep another two hours in the morning and again in the afternoon. After three days on the Total Multimune™ nutrients from Dr Brimhall, I awoke rested and feeling like a "real person" instead of a "sleeping beauty." I feel alert and have a lot more energy and am continuing on the Multimune supplement.

—Harriet

• • • • • • • • • • • • • • • • • • • •

SUMMARY

- The germ theory has distracted too much of the medical community into a narrow focus on drugs that offer only temporary relief.
- A nourished, exercised body and peaceful mind can resist infections.
- The natural flora in our GI tracts, when in the right balance, protects us from unfriendly bacteria, viruses and fungal yeasts.
- Just as weakened immune systems lower our defenses when we're depleted, an immune system strengthened by vitamins, minerals, herbs and other nutrients can assist our own immune systems to fight infections naturally and successfully.

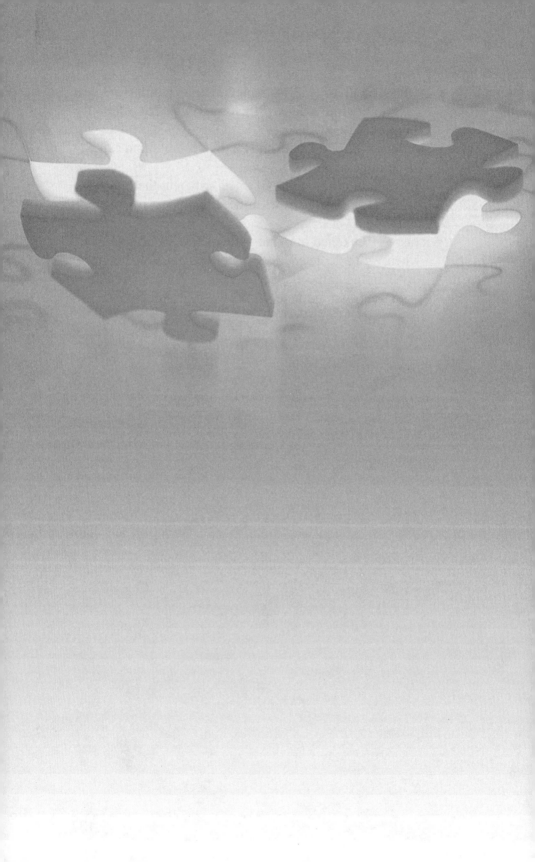

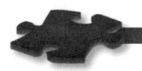

Step 3D
Replace Enzymes and/or HCL to Aid Digestion, Assimilation and Elimination

Now let's look at solutions for your human food processor – your digestive tract. Every system in the body can be positively affected by the electromagnetic energy in enzymes. Enzymes are living systems, living foods. Enzymes in raw foods electrify and energize your system even before they enter the digestive tract.

Enzymes protect the body from toxic waste byproducts by helping convert these wastes into forms that can be eliminated by the body. They can search out and help digest the body's own accumulated wastes, as well as the wastes left over from electromagnetic pollution.

COOKING AND ENZYMES

Most cooking leaves foods devoid of enzyme activity. If you look at the electromagnetic field of pasteurized milk versus raw milk, for example, the energy field of the pasteurized milk is virtually non-existent, while raw milk has a vibrant electromagnetic field. Supplemental enzymes help make up for enzymes destroyed in food preparation at temperatures above 118 degrees Fahrenheit.

LACK OF ENZYMES AND POOR DIGESTION

As a person ages, the body's production of hydrochloric acid and digestive enzymes declines, causing poor digestion. This leads to poor nutrition caused by a system that doesn't take in vitamins and minerals from food properly take in vitamins and minerals from food.

Partially undigested proteins can trigger allergies. Rheumatoid arthritis has been linked to food allergies and sensitivities. Proteolytic enzymes can reduce allergic symptoms. Once absorbed, protein-digesting enzymes can promote anti-inflammatory activity and may improve immune system function.

ACID REFLUX

Many people with acid reflux have low hydrochloric acid levels. Without enough acidity to signal the food to move on or to signal pancreatic enzymes to be secreted, the food sits and ferments in the stomach. There is nowhere to go but back up into the esophagus.

OTHER CAUSES OF POOR DIGESTION
- Poor dietary habits
- Hurrying through meals
- Gulping food
- Swallowing air
- Talking while chewing
- Drinking liquids with meals
- Overuse of antibiotics

ANTACIDS

Popular antacid medications aren't always a good solution; they neutralize necessary acids in the stomach, actually preventing proper digestion. Antacids interfere with nutrient absorption, making gas and bloating worse.

Poorly digested foods are linked with gas formation, heartburn and food allergies from undigested food particles.

Indigestion symptoms include:
- Gas
- Stomach pain
- Rumbling
- Bloating
- Belching
- Nausea
- Burning sensation

Poor digestion is also related to ulcers, bacterial colonization of the stomach, low stomach acid, low blood sugar and disorders of the gallbladder, liver and pancreas. Disappointment, worry, anxiety and stress can also interfere with healthy digestion.

● ● ● ● ● ● ● ● ● ● ● ● ● ● ● ● ● ● ● ●

A Case of Poor Digestion and Food Allergies
Dear Dr. Brimhall,

When I came to your office, my digestion was terrible. I had been eliminating more and more foods from my diet and adding more and more nutrients, to no avail. My energy was low, my heart was doing "flip-flops," and I had frequent headaches, neck pain and hot flashes (at age 65!) Also, my shoulder was frozen and I had overall stiffness. At your office, I was tested for allergies, had my blood analyzed, had nutrients kinetically tested to find out which ones my body wanted and had body and cranial work and chiropractic adjustments. I have followed the recommendations that I was given, and what a difference it has made! I am now feeling energetic, my heart is beating smoothly, I have far fewer headaches and my breathing is better. I am more limber and my frozen shoulder is loosening up. I am now able to eat a wide variety of foods (some I hadn't been able to eat for years) and am digesting them well. The hot flashes are greatly reduced. The recurring flu-like symptoms are gone. I look forward to continued improvement. This process allowed me to get well by freeing up my body's ability to restore health.
— Shirley K. B.

Total Enzymes™ (veg) provides a full spectrum of enzymes to aid digestion and assimilation.

ATTENTION DEFICIT DISORDER AND ADHD

Attention-deficit/hyperactivity disorder is a syndrome characterized by its descriptive name. Although it's often used to describe children who are inattentive, impulsive and hyperactive, 30-50% of those with ADHD in childhood manifest symptoms into adulthood.

Hyperactivity and Attention Deficit Disorder Characteristics

- Clumsiness
- Lack of concentration
- Learning disabilities
- Tendencies to disturb others
- Inability to finish tasks
- Difficulties in solving problems
- Low tolerance for stress
- Easily frustrated
- Sleep disturbances
- Failure in school
- Absent-mindedness
- Forgetfulness
- Self-destructiveness
- Mood swings
- Emotional instability
- Impatience
- Temper tantrums
- Hearing disorders
- Head-knocking
- Speech disorders
- Violence

Unfortunately, like many other syndromes, ADHD and related conditions have been treated for the symptoms, while the causes have not been addressed.

It is clear that poor digestion, nutritional deficiency, food additives, allergies, prescription drugs used to treat mental problems, mineral deficiencies, mineral ratios, heavy metals, electromagnetic stresses, physical illness, stress, environmental toxins and chemicals all play roles in causing ADHD.

One critical factor is nutritional deficiency, caused, in large part, by inadequate digestive enzymes and poor diet with inadequate protein. Other factors include: poor energy production by the cells or lack of proper mitochondria, smoking during pregnancy, pre-natal trauma, oxygen deprivation at birth, artificial food additives, and multiple allergies or sensitivities. Exposures to heavy metals such as lead and aluminum have also been linked to ADHD in some cases.

Patrick Sherry, the "Post Office Slayer," was found to have high levels of both cadmium and lead and a severe copper-zinc imbalance. James Huberty, the man who shot 24 people at a fast food restaurant, was found to have extremely high levels of cadmium. In people with childhood learning disabilities, high levels of copper, manganese, mercury, cadmium and lead have been found.

We use special methods to evaluate brain balance and use the Erchonia 635 nm laser to modulate activity. We have seen remarkable improvement in these conditions, when used in conjunction with the other steps to wellness.

YOU ARE WHAT YOU EAT

A diet regimen of organic, whole, natural foods, with emphasis on fresh, unprocessed foods, definitely helps. This includes all fruits and vegetables, with the exception of foods that contain salicylates, which are identified triggers of ADHD.

We've seen many reports of beneficial effects from a wholesome diet. Diets avoiding sugar, dairy, wheat, corn, chocolate and peanuts, along with artificial colors and preservatives, have been known to provide beneficial effects.

SUGAR AND ADHD

All refined sugars and products containing any of the many sugars must be avoided for those with ADHD. Sugar consumption is linked with abnormal blood sugar levels, which can trigger mood swings and other emotional problems.

ADHD sufferers should avoid all carbonated beverages that contain sugar or aspartame. Aspartame contains concentrated amounts of amino acids that affect brain chemistry. High levels of phosphorus normally mean low levels of magnesium and calcium, which can trigger both hyperactivity and seizures.

USE FOOD FOR THERAPY

In one study of thousands of children with ADHD, 53% were successfully treated using nutritional therapy. 34% percent showed some improvement, and only 13% showed no improvement at all.

These studies were accomplished by changing only nutrition. Therefore, evaluating all 6 Interferences to Health and correcting with all 6 Steps to Wellness can give you much greater success.

For a nutritional program to be successful, it must be tailor-made to each individual. Heavy metal and other toxin analyses must be done, nutrition must be planned for the individual, and treatment of food allergies/sensitivities must be completed for full recovery from ADHD.

NEUROTRANSMITTERS: OUR BEST STRESS DEFENSE

Neurotransmitters called epinephrine and norepinephrine, produced in the brain's adrenal medulla, are much lower in ADHD children. One way to help ensure you or your child gets all the helpful nutrition to build the neurochemicals the brain needs is to promote healthy digestion and to eat fresh, organic foods, free of pesticide and chemical residues.

William Walsh, PhD, found that when insufficient stomach acid was corrected and digestion normalized, people subject to delinquency, irritability and impulsiveness of ADHD had no further need for treatment. All the problems of ADHD may be related to the body's inability to take in and absorb the nourishment it needs to be well.

To put all of the pieces together for health, you can use Total Mitochondria™ to increase energy, Total 5 HTP™ to increase serotonin levels, Total Chelate™ to help detoxify, Total Flax™ and Total Brain™ for natural nutritional brain support, homeopathic metal detox, cranial and spinal adjusting, fascial release, Erchonia™ cold laser therapy, foot bath detox, emotional release techniques and far infrared sauna treatment. Now that is a mouthful! That is also exactly what we do every day to treat the person, instead of the named and blamed condition!

SUMMARY

- Many of the symptoms we suffer, and the conditions we are diagnosed with, are the result of improper nutrition. We aren't getting proper nutrients to our tissues, organs and systems.
- Even if we eat right, few of us have adequate enzymes and proper bowel flora. This gives us poor digestion, assimilation and elimination.
- Supplementing with Total Enzymes™ (plant enzymes) can electrify the body and aid in the proper digestion of carbohydrates, proteins and fats.
- Proper supplementation is necessary with high-grade synergistic nutrition, for many individuals, to bring them back into balance.

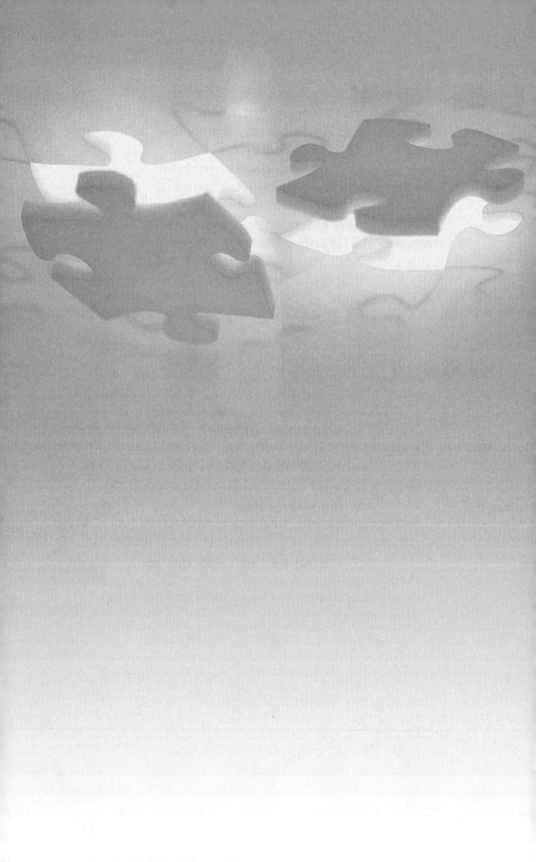

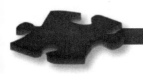

Step 3E
Restore Proper Bowel Flora to Optimize Colon Function

Poor digestion is often caused by a shortage of friendly bacteria. A fungal yeast infection (candida) sometimes complicates matters. Candida can be caused by oral antibiotic therapy, chemotherapy, oral contraceptives, corticosteroids, chlorinated water, heavy metal overloads, poor diet or underlying illnesses.

Supplemental probiotics help restore the normal balance of flora in the gastrointestinal (GI) tract and vagina and reduce candida overgrowth.

Poor digestion is often caused, not only by the overuse of antibiotics in health care, but also the overuse of antibiotics in raising animals for food. Antibiotics deplete and kill the friendly bacteria that normally inhabit the bowel along with harmful bacteria.

The ideal balance in the GI tract is at least 85% friendly bacteria and 15% coliform bacteria. In most people the balance is reversed, resulting in gas, bloating, intestinal and system-wide toxicity, malabsorption of nutrients and constipation. This imbalance also encourages the overgrowth of fungal yeast.

Probiotics can provide you with B Vitamins, Vitamin K and bacteriocin byproducts to inhibit the proliferation of unfriendly bacteria. Bacteriocins are also known to put lethal hits on cancer cells.

FOUR POUNDS OF GOOD GUYS

There are billions of bacteria in a healthy digestive tract. An estimated four pounds of these bacteria are friendly and help maintain good health. They produce the milk-digesting enzyme lactase and can inhibit or deactivate disease-causing bacteria, viruses and yeast, by starving or killing bad bacteria.

They play an important role in the development of a healthy immune system, preventing allergies and malabsorption problems. Good bacteria also protects against radiation and toxic pollutants while helping recycle estrogen.

In supplement therapy, friendly bacteria have been shown useful in treating acne, psoriasis, eczema, allergies, migraine, gout (by reducing uric acid levels), arthritic conditions, cystitis, candidiasis, irritable bowel and some forms of cancer.

Probiotic supplements are best taken on an empty stomach, away from mealtimes. Stomach acidity during meals can damage the cultures' viability. After opening a bottle, it's best stored in the refrigerator.

Poor digestion is also related to ulcers, unfriendly bacterial infection in the stomach, low stomach acid, low blood sugar and disorders of the gallbladder, liver and pancreas. Our favorite supplement to help re-establish bowel flora is Total Probiotics™.

WHO NEEDS A LEAKY GUT?

With contributions by Lynn Toohey, PhD
Nutri-West Researcher and Contributing Author

Newsweek magazine featured an article about tiny leaks in the lining of the small intestine that may play a role in diseases that range from asthma to arthritis.

This focuses new awareness on one of the oldest immune weapons we have – our own gut lining. The lining of our intestines are meant not only to absorb food, but also to act as a barrier to keep out invading pathogens.

The lining of a healthy gut filters out microorganisms and undigested proteins. When things like aspirin, bacteria or even the pesticides sprayed on our food batter this lining, the lining loses its integrity. This is when the door swings open to let in bacteria, viruses, parasites and undigested food particles, which can activate the immune system and also the autoimmune system. We refer to this loss of integrity as, "the leaky gut syndrome." It's not a pretty name, and not a pretty condition.

Symptoms related to leaky gut include: fatigue, arthritis pains, muscle pains, fever, stomach discomfort, diarrhea, skin rashes, memory problems and shortness of breath.

You need to protect the intestinal lining to keep your gut strong and disease-resistant. Healing the gut lining is important in such conditions as: asthma, arthritis, food allergies, ulcers, Crohn's disease, ulcerative colitis, celiac disease, autoimmune diseases, alcoholism, chronic fatigue, joint pain, migraines, diarrhea, parasite infections, dysbiosis, candidiasis, multiple sclerosis, diabetes and T-cell lymphomas.

People put themselves at risk for intestinal permeability and leakage if they:

- Smoke
- Drink
- Take aspirin or ibuprofen
- Take antibiotics or other drugs
- Are exposed to environmental toxins
- Have poor digestion, sluggish liver detoxification or stored toxins
- Have bacterial/microbial infections or inflammation.

Research shows there are nutrients that help maintain the integrity of the intestinal lining. We have combined them in one synergistic blend called Total Leaky Gut™.

• •

Cases Affecting the Whole Body
I began using Total Leaky Gut™ and Homocysteine Redux™ for many of my clients. Within six to eight weeks, the whole fiber structure of the iris began to change greatly. Where the fibers were wide and white, they were becoming narrower, and the white was decreasing. I am an Iridologist, and Iridology is a great tool to understanding the body's systems: these products have shown how homocysteine and a leaky gut affect the whole body.
— Dr. Hannah P.

• •

FRIENDLY FIBER

Fiber is important to maintaining regularity, but it's not the only answer. Many nutrients are responsible for maintaining the health and motility of the colon. Fiber is, however, one of the major players in determining the health of the colon.

The colon is a muscle and, just like any muscle, it needs to be exercised to be healthy. Fiber exercises the colon, preventing the formation of pouches that develop into diverticulosis.

In addition to exercising the colon, fiber helps maintain easy movement through the colon. Fiber also contributes to the consistency of the stool. Both soluble and insoluble fibers contribute to the health of the colon, and fibers are found in plant substances such as oats and apple pectin. Soluble fiber can regulate blood sugar by decreasing gastric emptying and glucose uptake. This reduces insulin response and fat storage.

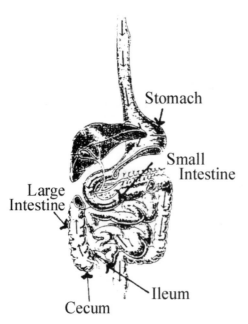

Stomach

Small Intestine

Large Intestine

Cecum

Ileum

THE NUTRIENTS YOU NEED

Probiotics: These build the immune system and contribute to the motility of the colon. Many times, constipation is relieved by restoring a healthy balance of flora to the large intestine. Different varieties of lactobacillus (i.e., acidophilus, casei, plantarum, rueteri, salicarius, etc.) and bifidobacteria (i.e. bifidum, longum) can play specific therapeutic roles in the colon. A healthy balance of good flora will produce Vitamin K and most of the B Vitamins.

Digestive Enzymes: Food needs to be broken down and assimilated; incomplete breakdown fosters fermentation and putrefaction. Undigested food impedes the healthy function of the colon. Plant enzymes work in a wide pH range, increasing their effectiveness along the entire GI tract. Amylase breaks down starch, protease breaks down protein, and lipase breaks down fat. Enzymes such as invertase, malt diastase and lactase can break down starch/sugars, while cellulase breaks down the fiber of plant cell walls.

L-Glutamine Plus™ (veg): Nutrient Formula for Colon Support and Rebuilding promotes healthy intestinal walls, normalizes GI pH, helps the body produce its own B Vitamins, provides the body with its own antibiotic defenses, discourages unfriendly microbes, and assists in healthy digestion.

SUMMARY

- The ideal balance in the GI tract is at least 85% of friendly bacteria and 15% of coliform bacteria.
- You can rebalance the bowel with pre- and probiotics.
- Four pounds of our bowel is composed of friendly bacteria that play an important role in the development of a healthy immune system.
- When our bowel is healthy, we take one more step towards wellness.
- You need to protect the intestinal lining against "leaky gut" to keep you strong and disease-resistant.

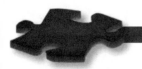

NUTRITION: EAT WELL TO BE WELL

An Addendum to Step 3

Amazingly, we humans know the importance of putting the right grade of gasoline in our cars and choosing the right food for our pets, yet often skip meals or fill our bodies with sugar, hydrogenated oils, soda and alcohol, not realizing the impact our food and drink choices have on our health. We then seek a doctor who can give us a cure-all pill or a surgery that can remove what we caused by our own poor diet. It's a "name and blame" game. We give diseases a name and list of symptoms so we can blame something, other than ourselves, for our illness or lack of health, when it's really a product of our own creation.

Surveys show that 20% of the U.S. population never eats vegetables, and 40% rarely consumes fruit or fruit juices. The most popular vegetable consumed in the U.S. is the potato – not as a whole potato, but as the nearly empty calories in french fries and potato chips. Another 80% never consumes whole grains or high-fiber foods.

The empty calories in sugar are almost universal, in nearly all processed foods, as a flavor and texture enhancer. Sugar is recommended in recipe books and used in fast foods. All forms of refined sugar interfere with the abilities of white blood cells to destroy unfriendly bacteria and lower immune system function. Sugar also depletes the body of other nutrients. Alcohol, a relative of sugar, also weakens a wide variety of immune responses.

Protective and nourishing nutrients and phytochemicals are found abundantly in whole fruits and vegetables, and yet these are the very foods avoided by most people. Fruit and vegetable consumption in population studies has been consistently shown to reduce the risk of many degenerative diseases including diabetes, heart disease and cancer.

The "5-a-Day for Better Health" program, sponsored by the National Cancer Institute (NCI), encourages the public to include more fruits and vegetables in their diet, at least five servings a day.

The standard American diet, which contains food grown in depleted soils, has left Americans deficient in many nutrients important to health. Crops are repeatedly raised on the same field, year after year, with only artificial fertilizer designed to increase yields, but not nutritional content.

In 1936, U.S. Senate Document #264 cited nutritional deficiencies caused by our depleted soils. It also stated that 95% of Americans were deficient in one or more major minerals, and many trace minerals, that have proven to be necessary for bone mineralization.

One can only imagine how much further depletion has taken place since 1936. Contributing to this depletion, the standard American diet consisting of high sodium, high protein, high sugar, soft drinks, caffeinated beverages and processed foods leads to further mineral loss.

The National Academy of Medicine estimates that 15% of the U.S. population suffers from fatigue associated with chemical sensitivities (sometimes called Multiple Chemical Sensitivities). Many experts believe that a major cause of these problems stems from the post-World War II chemical revolution that put some 3,000 chemicals in our foods, 700 chemicals in our drinking water, and another 10,000 in food processing and storage. The EPA has found over 400 toxic chemicals in human tissue associated with fatigue, depression, mental, motor and neurological disorders, and cancer. Over 81 drugs listed in the Physicians Desk Reference have "chronic fatigue" as a known side effect. Additionally, cooking, food processing and microwaving all take their toll on creating nutritional deficiencies.

SO, WHAT DO WE DO NOW?

The solution is to choose whole, organic foods grown by natural means on replenished soils. At all costs, avoid empty foods that deplete your body.

Do

- Shop in the fresh-foods aisles
- Eat fresh meats, fish and produce
- Choose organic and natural foods
- Eat 5 to 8 servings of natural, fresh vegetables a day
- Eat fresh, whole potatoes
- Drink 8 to 10 glasses of pure water to assist toxin removal

Don't

- Shop in the canned-foods aisles
- Eat fried foods
- Drink soft drinks
- Eat canned foods
- Eat convenience or junk foods
- Eat bakery goods
- Eat margarine or any hydrogenated fat
- Drink caffeinated drinks
- Drink alcohol to excess

You can rebuild your body and immune system with natural, whole foods, and you can take good supplements to help replenish the nutrients necessary to rebuild your organs, glands and systems. When the body's systems are working at 100%, you have 100% wellness. Eat well to be well.

GOOD FATS VS. BAD FATS

Richard Passwater was one of the first to set the record straight on fats and cholesterol. Believe it or not, fats and cholesterol in the diet are good for you!

Passwater found population studies comparing vegetarian monks to those who consumed meat, cream and butter. Both groups showed equal rates of heart disease. This suggested that whatever caused heart disease was not related to fat and cholesterol consumption.

Similar population studies showed that African tribes who consumed enormous quantities of meat, fat and cholesterol had no greater rates of heart disease than other tribes who were strictly vegetarian.

If that's not enough to suggest that fat and cholesterol aren't bad for you, consider the studies of 500 Irish twin brothers. Half of the twins remained in Ireland and ate a diet high in meat, eggs, bacon and fatback, while the other half emigrated to New York City, where they ate diets high in processed foods. The brothers remaining in Ireland with high-fat diets showed hearts that appeared years younger than their city counterparts! The processed foods with empty calories and damaged fats, in the city, were the evil nemesis.

As Dr. Zane Kime, and others, point out, many studies show increased rates of heart disease and cancer from high fat consumption. But, as Dr. Kime correctly suspected, many of the studies didn't inquire into the quality of fat and cholesterol consumed. His suspicions led him to believe that it was trans fats that were the actual cause of statistics linking fat to disease.

● ● ● ● ● ● ● ● ● ● ● ● ● ● ● ● ● ● ● ●

Processed Foods (Don't Eat!)
- White Breads
- Crackers
- Pastries
- Baked goods
- Cake/Frosting mixes
- Doughnuts
- Baking mixes
- Processed sauces
- Frozen vegetables
- Frozen dinners
- Canned soups
- Breakfast cereals

● ● ● ● ● ● ● ● ● ● ● ● ● ● ● ● ● ● ●

Trans fats are partially hydrogenated vegetable oils found commonly in all processed foods. Even health food stores carry processed foods with trans fats, so read labels!

In Puerto Rico, breast and colon cancer rates are only 30-40% of the rates in the United States, yet Puerto Rican diets are composed of 88% animal fat. Americans, on the other hand, consume most of their fats in artificially tinkered-with, overheated, chemically damaged vegetable fats ... or trans fats.

Trans fats are created in the refining process when polyunsaturated fats are removed from food sources. During this process, the polyunsaturated fats are deodorized, and their molecular structure changes from their natural horseshoe shape to a straight-line structure.

Our body's cells attempt to use this artificial fat, but the DNA blueprint calls for the horseshoe shape. The results are that holes are created in the cell walls, and debris begins to collect inside cells. Also, the salt concentration increases within cell walls, and the energy furnaces of the cells swell to two or three times their normal size!

Human cells, on the standard American diet, contain up to 14% of these trans fats. As the concentration of artificial fats increases in the cell, the cells not only swell, but their energy functions and building and repair functions are damaged, setting the stage for disease processes.

Conventionally created, processed "pure" liquid oils have about 6% trans fats. Margarine contains about 54%, and solid vegetable shortening (fully hydrogenated oils) contains as much as 58% trans fats. These are produced by food manufacturing companies. Please know that trans fats are deadly.

It's rare to find a label anywhere that doesn't proudly claim that its processed food is "low in fat and cholesterol." This fat that is in processed, canned and packaged foods can't be natural fat without the risk of spoilage ... which means it's usually trans fat.

EAT FATS TO BE HEALTHY

Dr. Diana Schwarzbein's work has made the health value of natural, undamaged fats very clear. Fats and cholesterol don't cause heart disease. You must eat good fats to <u>prevent</u> heart disease.

Eating good fats allows you to be healthy. Cholesterol is a kind of fat that is essential to maintain the membranes of all cells. Good dietary cholesterol is necessary for the body to build its hormones, including sex and adrenal hormones.

Cholesterol is necessary for cell growth, the nervous system and healthy brain function. Don't eat good fats, and you will starve your brain.

EMOTIONAL DISORDERS AND FATS

Replenishing fats has been important in reversing ADD, and helpful in other disorders, such as, schizophrenia. As Dr. Schwarzbein points out, many instances of depression, agitation and irritability can be caused by insufficient intake of good fats. Good fats are essential to healthy brain function. They're necessary to stabilize moods. The brain's dry weight is composed of 70% cholesterol! The myelin sheath requires cholesterol to insulate our nerves.

● ● ● ● ● ● ● ● ● ● ● ● ● ● ● ● ● ●

Sources of Natural Cholesterol and Fat

- Eggs
- Butter
- Cream
- Sour cream
- Raw milk
- Raw cheeses
- Nuts
- Seeds
- Nut butters
- Seed butters
- Red meat
- Chicken
- Shellfish
- Avocados (80% fat)
- Olives
- Tofu
- Cold-pressed olive oil

- Extra-virgin olive oil (pure-pressed or expeller-pressed oils are best from plant sources)

Your body needs good fats from both plant and animal sources. Saturated, monounsaturated and polyunsaturated fats are all good for you! Your diet should be rich in fat and cholesterol from a variety of foods.

When you don't get an adequate amount of fat, you become subject to emotional disorders, insomnia, allergies, asthma, brittle nails, scaly and itchy skin, dry, limp and thinning hair, joint pain, infertility, acid reflux, constipation, carbohydrate cravings, and other problems.

COOKING DAMAGES FATS

Heat does damage to animal fat. French fries, potato chips and all other deep-fried foods should be avoided as well: they're made with damaged fats. All damaged fats harm the cells of the body, producing cellular debris and causing accelerated aging of all cells.

The lower the temperature in cooking meat and fish, the better. The blackened parts of steak and roasts are damaged fat caused by high-temperature cooking. Heat, in processing conventional vegetable oils, also damages liquid vegetable oils.

The natural oil in whole corn is good for you; the heat and chemically processed stuff in conventional oils is bad for you. All chemically and heat-processed oils outside of a health food store, with the exception of extra-virgin olive oil, should be avoided. Anything in the label that says partially hydrogenated or hydrogenated is pure poison.

For salad dressings, use corn, cottonseed, poppy seed, safflower, sesame, soybean, sunflower and walnut oils, as long as they're pure-pressed, not heat processed or chemically processed. If they're expeller-pressed (good for you), it says so on the label. If it doesn't say so, don't buy it, and don't eat it.

All of these oils and cooking oils should be refrigerated after opening, because the air can damage them through oxidation, just as high-temperature cooking damages oils by oxidation. Never over-charbroil. Low, slow cooking is best. Medium rare is better than well done.

Good oils for cooking are butter, coconut, avocado, canola, mustard, olive, peanut, almond and rice oil. Use real cream, and real butter because homogenized and pasteurized milk products such as half-and-half contain damaged fats.

OMEGA-3 FATTY ACIDS

Although not appropriate for cooking, fish oil is a rich source of omega-3 fatty acids, EPA and DHA. To a limited extent, flaxseed oil converts into EPA. Omega-3s are good for you on many levels. They have blood-thinning effects, keep blood triglycerides in check and have anti-inflammatory benefits. They're found abundantly in such ocean-run fish as salmon, mackerel, herring, sardines, black cod, anchovies and albacore tuna. They're also found in wild game, free-range eggs and grass-fed beef.

LOW-FAT AND LOW-CALORIE DIETS

Carbohydrates are sugars, either simple or complex. Hi-protein/low-complex carbohydrate diets promoted for weight loss are effective; however, the weight loss is from muscle at the expense of added body fat. That's why these diets are so popular. Muscle weighs more, so the scales tell you you've lost weight. You have. You've lost muscle weight, while becoming fatter.

When too many sugars are consumed, which is common with diet candy bars, diet drinks or diets that emphasize simple-carbohydrate meals (starchy vegetables, pasta and bread), too much insulin is released. When too many carbs are consumed, insulin tells the liver to increase fat production from the incoming sugar.

The good news is that insulin helps replenish and refuel cells and helps keep blood sugar levels balanced. However, only protein foods tell the pancreas to release glucagon as well as insulin. Glucagon is not released when non-starchy vegetables or fats are eaten. When glucagon levels are high in ratio to insulin (a response to protein eating), glucagon tells the cells to burn fat as fuel and to use food for building and repair. If only protein is eaten, the insulin to glucagon ratio is too low.

THE PERFECT MEAL

The perfect meal is always composed of a balance of proteins, fats, non-starchy vegetables and complex carbohydrates. When you eat processed carbs, such as refined grains or white bread, you have a rapid rise in insulin. When whole starchy vegetables, like whole potatoes or carrots, are eaten (complex carbohydrates), less insulin is secreted, but this level will still be too high if these foods are eaten alone.

When you eat a balanced meal (maybe steak, baked sweet potato, butter and vegetables with a salad), digestion is slowed down, and the pancreas secretes a balanced level of glucagon and insulin.

Simple sugars enter the bloodstream fastest as they have a higher glycemic index. Complex carbohydrates contain fiber and complex sugars which slow the rate of sugar entering the bloodstream. They have a lower glycemic index. However, if you eat potatoes by themselves, the glycemic index of the complex carbohydrates will make the body store the excess calories as fat. When you combine a potato with meat, chicken, fish or soy protein, the ratio will be balanced. The balance of insulin and glucagon won't signal the body to store fat, but instead a balanced food meal will signal the body to make energy and build and repair the body. It's that simple.

• •

The Perfect Meal
Protein: fish, chicken, tofu, eggs or cheeses
Starchy Carbohydrate: potato, brown rice, corn, carrots,whole grains or sprouted grain bread,
Fat: butter, sour cream, olive oil, corn oil, sunflower oil or nuts,
Non-Starchy Carbohydrate: lettuces, broccoli, zucchini, cauliflower or bell peppers,

• •

PROTEIN

How much? If your activity levels are high, eat more protein. If you are sedentary, eat much less. And of course, do common-sense adjustments for your size and weight. Generally, the minimum amount of protein you should eat ranges from 2 to 5 ounces, and about 1 to 3 ounces for a snack.

VEGETABLES

I Eat non-starchy vegetables with every meal. They're rich in antioxidants, vitamins, minerals and protective phytonutrients that protect against all major diseases. Five to eight servings is the best choice.

FRUIT

Fruit should never be eaten by itself because it raises insulin levels too high. It should <u>always</u> be eaten with healthy fats and protein, ideally with the fully balanced meal of protein, fat, carbohydrate and vegetables.

CARBOHYDRATES OR STARCHY FOODS

The general rule for minimum intake of complex carbohydrates (whole foods, not refined sugar) is 15 grams with each meal, which is slightly more than 1/2 an ounce.

They are poisons. If you have a sugar craving, satisfy it with whole fruit, and balance it with protein, fat and vegetables.

STRESS

Under stressful conditions, simply eat less. Stress interferes with digestion. Stress also raises adrenalin and cortisol levels <u>unless</u> you eat more moderately and frequently than usual. So, eat smaller, balanced meals under stressful conditions.

People experiencing stress develop carb cravings because stress depletes serotonin levels, and carbs raise serotonin levels. (See Step 3 A-E for supplements that enhance healthy function). Ideally, you should take supplementary digestive enzymes with each meal, unless it's a raw food meal or snack. Also take friendly flora supplements between meals to make the most of the food that you do eat and to re-establish proper intestinal flora.

SAMPLE BALANCED MEALS

How much of what? Rather than measure grams or ounces, use your plate as your measuring device. One-third of the plate should be protein, one-third should be carbohydrate, and the last third should be vegetables. Then add good, non-processed fats to the carb portion such as butter or good extra-virgin olive oil or another cold-pressed oil to the salad or the vegetable.

Ideally, three small balanced meals per day and two snacks should be eaten. If not, three balanced meals. Never skip meals. Fasting one meal will interfere with insulin levels at the next meal.

Coffee should be avoided, since it raises hormone levels. Caffeinated beverages and alcohol deplete necessary vitamins and minerals. Green and black or herbal teas are better, or water with lemon. Never drink carbonated drinks. If alcohol is consumed, it should be moderate. If you want milk, drink raw milk.

Again, never deep fry, and never over-charbroil. Also, never microwave. Microwaving makes foods toxic, destroys nutrients, and makes you fat. Drink plenty of pure water between meals, before meals, and after meals, but not with meals.

These are samples only. They're not meant to restrict your choices in proteins, carbohydrates or vegetables. Be creative and follow your individual taste. Eat whole, unprocessed, organic foods where possible, and always use fresh meats, fruits and vegetables.

SNACKS

The ideal is to combine a carb with protein at each snack.

BREAKFAST

1/3 of plate: egg(s), spinach-mushroom omelet cooked with

butter, red meat, fish, tofu or cheeses.

1/3 of plate: sprouted grain or organic whole grain toast with butter, seed or nut butters, or granola.

1/3 of plate: fruits, like blueberries, banana or apple slices.

SNACK

A handful of raw nuts, nut or seed butter with an apple; 1/4 to 1/2 cup of blueberries with a piece of cheese; four sticks of celery with peanut butter; or 1/4 to 1/2 cup of yogurt with same amount of strawberries, cherries, etc.

LUNCH

1/3 of the plate: fish, calamari, shrimp, lobster, oysters or clams.

1/3 of the plate: organic brown rice, wild rice, or baked or mashed potato with butter and sour cream.

1/3 of the plate: broccoli, cauliflower, Brussels sprouts, or your choice of a non-starchy veggie.

SNACK

1/4 cup sunflower seeds; 1 1/2 tablespoons of cashews or almonds; or 1/4 cup cottage cheese with 1/4 to half a cup of fresh fruit.

DINNER

1/3 of plate: natural steak, lamb chops, turkey, chicken, game, organic cheeses or pork.

1/3 of plate: an ear of organic corn with real butter, carrots or potato.

1/3 of the plate: mixed green salad, tomatoes, bell peppers, onions, with extra-virgin olive oil, sunflower or walnut oil, or fresh lemon juice.

SUMMARY

- Poor diets interfere with the body's ability to nourish, rebuild and heal itself.
- Stay out of the center of supermarkets.
- Shop in the outside aisles for fresh fruits, vegetables, raw cheeses, raw milk and fresh meats and seafood.
- Eat organic nourishing foods grown on rich soils.
- Avoid junk foods, bakery goods, processed foods, canned or frozen foods, soft drinks and sugar.
- Nutrients can help repair all of our glands, organs, muscles and tissues.
- Hearts and arteries, weakened by improper diet and lifestyle, can be strengthened, fit and well.
- The body has all it needs to rebuild and repair itself nutritionally.

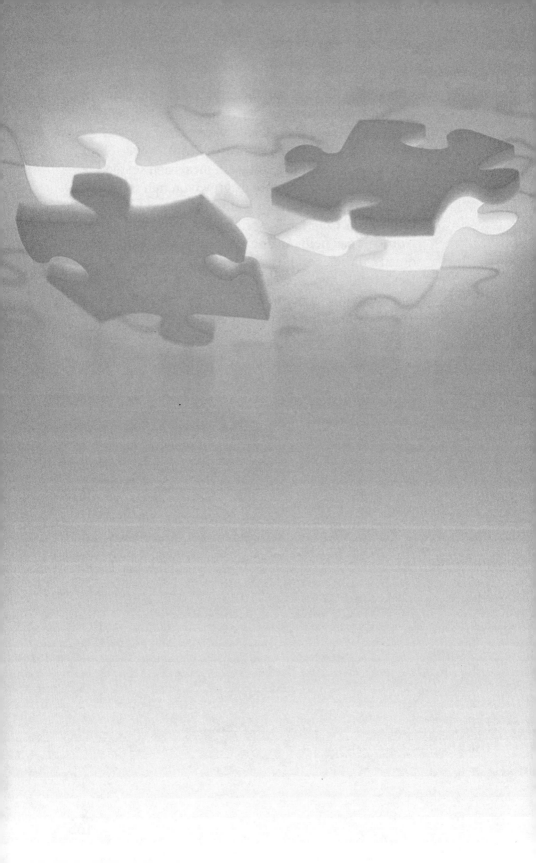

REPROGRAM THE BODY FOR ALLERGIES/SENSITIVITIES

An allergy is the body's abnormal reaction to a substance, or group of substances, which a healthy body would consider harmless. This reaction will cause an abnormal physical response to the substance, known as an allergen or an antigen, the substance may be toxic to everyone. These may include: exhaust fumes, petrochemicals or pesticides – or it may be as innocent as a common food or smell.

When the body is exposed to these substances, it may trigger an excess of an antibody called immunoglobulin E (this is termed an IgE-mediated response). Histamines are released from cell tissues, producing various symptoms.

The body can also become oversensitive to any substance and react as if it's being invaded. The body might mobilize its defense mechanisms even if a true IgE response can't be measured. We refer to this as "sensitivity," rather than a true allergy, although both can yield the same kinds of symptoms and reactions.

We believe almost every serious condition can have an allergic component, including:

- Addictions
- Asthma
- Arthritis
- Acne
- Back pain
- Diarrhea
- Depression
- Candida/yeast infections
- Colitis
- Constipation
- Eczema

- Flatulence/GERD
- Hay fever
- Headaches
- Hyperactivity
- Insomnia
- Indigestion
- Migraines
- Sinusitis
- Weight problems
- Vertigo

Studies show that at least 35 million people in the U.S. suffer from allergies. Many practitioners who deal with allergies believe the number is much higher and that most people suffer from some kind of allergy.

Allergies/sensitivities can be triggered by inhalants, ingestants, contactants, injectants or infectants. Most allergies are caused by a substance in the environment or by foods or food additives.

Reactions to allergens could include coughing, wheezing, itching, runny eyes, runny nose, hives and skin rashes, headache and fatigue or a colon spasm, etc. Allergy reactions can also mimic a wide range of diseases and disorders as previously listed.

To evaluate allergies and sensitivities, your physician may look at your personal history combined with physical examination, muscle response tests, skin response tests, blood tests, etc.

ATTACK OF THE MOLD SPORES

Mold is one of the most common environmental allergens. Molds are microscopic living organisms that love dark and damp places. They thrive in the air, soil, dead leaves, other organic material, and on some foods such as melons.

Mold spores are distributed by the wind and are problematic year-round in warm climates, and in the summer and early fall in other climates. You might provoke allergic reactions by walking through vegetation, cutting grass or repairing old furniture.

You can reduce the number of mold spores in your house by installing incandescent lights in dark closets and under sinks, and by disinfecting walls, basements, refrigerators and bathrooms.

It's also helpful to install electronic filtration systems, or use paper filters, in furnaces and air conditioners that trap mold, dust, pollen and bacteria. Commonly available ionic air purifiers can take many allergens out of the air.

WHY DO YOU SNEEZE, ETC.?

The immune system overreacts to substances it considers as invaders. How is it that the immune system gets into this overdrive gear and produces adverse immune system reactions? Many causes have been identified. One is that the immune system is overstressed by an overload of toxins: heavy metals accumulation (See Step 6), electromagnetic pollution (See Step 2) or pollution from air, water and food.

Some researchers feel that infant immune systems are damaged by too many vaccinations administered before the immune system has matured. In Japan, no vaccination is allowed before a child reaches 2 years of age because of the immaturity of the immune system, which needs exposure to many common irritants and childhood infectious processes in order to mature properly.

Other reasons your immune system might overreact are the overuse of antibiotics, fungal yeast infectants, virus, bacteria and parasite infectants, poor digestion, enzyme deficiencies, magnesium deficiencies, vitamin deficiencies, birth control pills, over-the-counter pain killers, steroids or heredity.

IS YOUR IMMUNE SYSTEM CONFUSED?

Antibiotic overuse leads to confused immune system responses. When antibiotics are used as routinely as penicillin (the miracle cure for everything and everyone during the early 20th century), the immune system eventually confuses the antibiotic with a foreign invader, and can no longer tell the difference between what is self and not self. Penicillin has now become one of the most common drugs to cause allergic reactions. It's also the most common antibiotic fed to livestock – not to treat infections, but to prevent them from more weight gain.

After the immune system has been stressed and confused, it begins to react to all kinds of harmless substances, as if they were enemies to the body. Bacteria, virus and parasite remnants can also remain in the bodies of people prone to allergies and asthma, bonding with tissues in the lungs, triggering inflammation, recurrent cycles of infection and allergic reactions.

• •

A Case History of Asthma

Health Condition: 15-year-old boy with lifelong asthma. Scar tissue in the lungs was so bad that doctors thought the boy had pneumonia when looking at his x-rays. Even with the best drugs, the boy had to use an inhaler an average of 5 times per day, and he had to be on oxygen at night. Even on oxygen, his blood oxygen level was no higher than 92%; normal should be 98-99%.

Comments: Using the *6 Steps To Wellness*, including A/SERT, gradually brought the times he used the inhaler down to 2 times a day within about 5 treatments. He needed daily Homocysteine Redux™ and Virx™ tablets for nutritional support. On the sixth visit, the percussor was used over his rib cage and lung, from which he noticed an immediate improvement in his breathing. He has not needed an inhaler since then, for the past week.

— Dr. Alvin B., DC
Brimhall Certified Practitioner

• •

DON'T KILL YOUR FRIENDS

Antibiotics can also kill off the friendly protective bacteria in our GI tracts, which encourages fungal yeast infection as well as viral and bacterial infections.

These kinds of infective organisms are linked with leaky gut syndrome or excessive permeability of the GI tract, partly caused by damaged walls in the digestive tract that allow food particles into the bloodstream.

The causes of a leaky gut include poor digestion, oral antibiotics, candida infection, viral, bacterial, and parasite infestations, alcohol consumption, over-the-counter painkillers, premature birth, the use of birth control pills and radiation.

Food in the digestive tract is normal, but food particles in the bloodstream are reacted to as foreign invaders. After the immune system reacts to food in the bloodstream, eating becomes a problem, sometimes leading to food intolerance.

We use a combination of pre- and probiotics we formulated called Total Probiotics™. We have formulated a combination of pre- and probiotics called Total ProbioticsTM for such conditions. Balanced bowel flora helps digest food, produce B Vitamins and Vitamin K, discourage viral and bacterial infections, prevent fungal yeast infection and reduce bloating. Friendly flora also produces lactase (the milk-digesting enzyme), which will allow those who are intolerant or allergic to dairy products to digest them without problems (See Step 3E for further information).

HOW FOOD CAN HARM YOU

Remnants of undigested food particles can cause allergic reactions. Any partially digested protein, carbohydrate or fat particle that enters the bloodstream will be recognized by the immune system as a foreign invader and treated as an allergen.

We always recommend that people, subject to allergies, chew their food slowly and completely to begin a healthy digestive process. We also test for enzymes that strengthen you when allergies have been identified. There's no better insurance than taking a full set of digestive enzymes with meals to make sure that proteins, carbohydrates and fats are digested fully and broken down completely so they won't enter the bloodstream as allergens.

We also recommend taking digestive enzymes on an empty stomach, in addition to taking them with food, so enzymes can enter the rest of the body and find the remnants of circulating immune complexes, whether they're composed of food particles and immune complexes, or remnants of byproducts from old infections and immune complexes. Both of these can irritate tissues, weaken lungs and set you up for rounds of recurrent infections and allergic reactions.

Most people with allergies are deficient in amylase, a

carbohydrate- and sugar-digesting enzyme. Without fully digested carbs, undigested carbohydrate particles can become allergens themselves.

Amylase is known as an important natural anti-inflammatory that helps you fight against any allergen irritating your system. Sometimes people are deficient in this enzyme because they're allergic to it – the very enzyme that will help them. When this happens, desensitizing the person by reprogramming the immune system to recognize this allergen as a friendly helper, may be the only solution.

Protein-digesting enzymes, called proteases, are essential for healthy protein digestion and fighting allergies. Proteases help remove irritating tissue debris of circulating immune complexes, help repair and regenerate damaged tissues, and help break down foreign substances that the immune system might identify as allergens.

Protein-digesting enzymes are also natural anti-inflammatory agents and natural antibiotics that prevent infection by digesting the protein coatings of viruses, bacteria and other unfriendly organisms before they can grow into disease-causing populations. We test for deficiencies in protein-digesting enzymes because vulnerability to infections and poor digestion can be caused by protease deficiency.

Many people who have been taking drugs, like cortisone inhalers and prednisone, have lowered immune-system function, one of the common side effects of that class of drugs. With a weakened immune system, your resistance to infection declines, setting you up for bronchial and sinus infections typical of asthma and allergy sufferers.

So you can see why We use Total Enzymes™ from a plant source that contains protein, fat and carbohydrate digesting enzymes in one capsule. Allergic symptoms may improve as digestion improves and infectious byproducts and inflammation decline.

WHEN THE BODY ATTACKS ITSELF

Healthy kidneys, bowel, stomach, liver, lungs, immune system and skin are essential for the body to eliminate its own waste products, as well as the toxins to which it is exposed. Dr. Fulford taught that we eliminate 3% of our wastes by the bowel, 7% by urine, 20% by the skin, and 70% by breathing and exhaled water vapor.

In the healthy body, the immune system works very well to

172

identify foreign substances, binds with them and breaks them down into non-toxic forms for elimination from the body. The immune system recognizes foreign substances, and then attacks them with macrophages, which digest and degrade them for removal from the body.

In an allergic individual, however, an overload of toxic waste products and circulating immune complexes bind with tissues of the body, especially in the lungs, sinuses and skin — the places where allergic reactions most noticeably take place. When this overload happens, allergies rear their ugly heads manifest.

The immune system calls on its backup resources, causing the body to attack itself because the immune complexes are bound to, and confused with, its own tissues.

This constant attacking of the body's own tissues and organs can lead to a host of secondary degenerative disorders like Rheumatoid Arthritis (when the body attacks its own joints and related tissues), disorders in the thyroid (when the body attacks the thyroid) and asthma (when the body attacks the airways), etc.

Recreational drugs, corticosteroid inhalers, prednisone, alcohol and sugar can lower immune-system health, and macrophages stop doing their jobs to digest and remove the debris. The result is an overloaded body, overloaded and malfunctioning liver, and many allergic complications.

Part of the solution is to repair excretion and elimination functions of the body. Supplying digestive enzymes and digestive nutrients and rebalancing the bowel with proper flora can help accomplish this.

To ensure the kidneys and urine excretion functions are working well, you must increase your drinking of pure filtered water. You must also give up highly toxic foods and drinks containing alcohol, sugar, caffeine and excess salt. Avoid milk, chocolate, hydrogenated oils and fried foods, all of which toxify the body. You must choose whole, organic high-fiber foods that help with elimination through the bowel.

SORRY, YOUR BACK IS OUT NOW

Respiratory ailments, asthma and allergies have been linked with spinal misalignments. Children with asthma have shown an overall improvement in lung function after only 15 chiropractic alignments of the spine. Direct connections between spinal nerves and the respiratory system can affect lung health. In addition, misalignments in the neck and upper back produce muscle spasms that affect elimination of toxins through the lymph.

With a blocked lymphatic system, your body's waste products, bacterial debris and toxins accumulate in lungs and other areas subject to allergy and asthma symptoms.

In many cases, chiropractic adjusting produces immediate relief of neck and back muscle stiffness, enhances circulation of the lymph and blood, and improves immune function, breathing and elimination of toxic materials. When spinal adjustment is combined with other therapies like allergy desensitization through A/SERT, you see even faster relief from allergy suffering.

SELF-HELP FOR ALLERGIES

Skin Brushing: Buy a vegetable brush at a health foods store. Brush your skin toward the heart for five minutes before bathing or showering. This helps increase blood and lymph circulation to the skin, the largest detoxification organ on the human body.

Salt and Soda Baths: Put 1-2 cups of Epsom salts and 1 cup baking soda in a tub of water and soak for 20-30 minutes (longer than that may cause fatigue). These baths can be taken two to three times per week and can help with allergies, pain, fatigue and many other conditions (other types of baths are detailed in Step 6).

VARY AND ROTATE YOUR DIET

Diets of allergy patients are normally repetitive and monotonous, consisting of 30 processed foods or less, filled with food chemicals and additives, which are eaten again and again.

One of the best things you can do for yourself is to avoid canned, processed and prepared conventional foods and choose natural, organic foods instead. In making this choice, you will have removed the entire chemical pollution associated with food intolerances and allergies and begin to nourish your system with healthy food.

Second, eat a variety of fresh, whole foods. Variety will not only reduce allergic reactions, but may help you lose a few extra pounds, just by choosing a range of different foods.

If you eat a wheat product like bread one day, don't eat another wheat product for several days. This is known as food rotation. Even if a food produces an adverse immune system reaction, the reaction will be minimal with food rotation.

Nutrients that support the immune system, including Vitamin A and zinc, can enhance the amount of an immune-system antibody production called IgA. It engulfs foreign matter so it won't be absorbed into the bloodstream.

A/SERT (Allergy/Sensitivity Elimination and Reprogramming Technique)

Identifying problematic or potentially allergic foods can be done much faster and more completely in a practitioner's office with muscle response testing, where one or a group of foods can be tested at a time.

The value of the clinically administered A/SERT technique is that it's fast and often a permanent way to desensitize your body to allergenic foods, substances and allergens. This procedure frees you of many allergies, pains and symptoms you had no idea could be helped.

ASKING THE BODY QUESTIONS

Kinesiology, or muscle response testing, is gaining broad recognition as a valuable diagnostic tool in the field of holistic or wellness health care. We use kinesiology to ask the body questions.

Just as a computer is programmed and communicates in a binary language, so does the body communicate in this yes-no fashion. If you ask a person a question and test a muscle that's strong, and the person answers truthfully, the muscle will remain strong. But if the person lies when tested, a previously strong muscle will weaken.

By the same token, when you introduce a substance that's good for a person, they will remain strong when tested. If a substance is ingested or even placed in the hand of a person who is allergic or sensitive to it, his or her muscles will weaken when tested.

Everything we eat, or come in contact with, has either a positive or negative effect on us. In fact, every thought we have or act we commit has a positive or negative stimulus on our nervous system, is recorded in the body and can be tested with kinesiology.

We can easily test foods, or vials containing foods, and see if they make you strong or weak. If they weaken you, we use a series of steps to rewrite the body's program so these substances no longer compromise your immune system.

We also use color and sound vibration to identify organs and systems involved, as well as help overcome emotional and physical problems. The cold laser can also be tuned to help reprogram the body and mind and eliminate sensitivities or allergenic problems. Structural adjustment and the meridian system are also used to reprogram the body.

WHAT IS A/SERT?

Allergy/Sensitivity Elimination and Reprogramming Technique is a specific protocol to rewrite the script in the body, so it no longer reacts to the allergens or similar substances as it did before. We *identify* the offending substance, *eliminate* it temporarily and *reprogram* the body. Many times this is permanent and gives the person a whole new lease on life.

The following is a simplified summary of deep clearing for a patient in our clinical setting:

The patient holds a food or substance or a vial containing a chemical, food, homeopathic, toxic metal or organ substance that causes muscle weakness. This is like pulling up on your computer screen what you want to work on. During this procedure, a spinal, acupressure/acupuncture/energy balance and brain balance is accomplished with the Erchonia Adjustor, Percussor and 635 nm laser. These adjuncts are used to harmonize weak and problematic areas and clear any energy, circulation, fascia, muscle, lymphatic or other restrictions. This deletes (in computer terms) and rewrites the script where the body responds to the substance differently and removes the aberrant reaction.

Color or sound therapy may also be used to help re-establish coherent communication for the body yielding healthy balance or central integration of the nervous system. Once the body, has been reprogrammed, the information is locked in through specific points along the meridian system. The cold laser or acupuncture sparkers are used to stimulate, in a clockwise circle, acupuncture points from the right hand around the body down the leg and up the other side, ending back on the right hand.

When completed with the A/SERT full cycle, the held allergen substance will no longer weaken the patient. Each clearing process for the allergen or allergens can take up to 15 to 20 minutes. With these advanced techniques, using the 635 nm Erchonia cold laser and specific nutritional support, it may take less than 20 minutes to complete the process in most cases.

It is recommended that the treated person avoid the substance(s) they were desensitized to for 25 hours. That's one 24-hour acupuncture cycle plus one hour for a safety margin.

HISTORY AND MANUAL ALLERGY TECHNIQUES

Dr. Devi Nambudripad is given credit for much of the research and development of manual allergy techniques. Dr. Nambudripad had allergic reactions to nearly every food, except rice and broccoli. One day, she absentmindedly ate a few pieces of a carrot while waiting for her rice to cook and her broccoli to steam. In only a few minutes, she had an allergic reaction and was about to pass out. She called her husband and asked for her acupuncture needles, performed a self-treatment by inserting the needles and then passed out.

Dr. Nambudripad slept for 45 minutes and awoke feeling very different, with high energy instead of the sick-and-tired feeling she normally got after an allergic reaction. She looked down to see some of the carrots in her hand, and some were on the bed where she had been lying on them. Her brain and body had been reprogrammed by treating while the allergic substance was in her energy field.

This wonderful accident led her to experiments that resulted in the Nambudripad Allergy Elimination Technique (NAET). When she treated herself for other foods she was allergic to, in a similar fashion, each food allergy disappeared. She has trained many therapists to use NAET.

A/SERT is our creative reformulation of this original breakthrough that, through years of use, has become more and more successful for fast reprogramming of the body to reduce or remove allergies and sensitivities.

The reason A/SERT works can be explained by biophysics and acupuncture theory. Everything has an electromagnetic field. When the brain interprets something as a threat to the body – for example, the electromagnetic field of a metal, food, contactant or pollen – the brain and body develop a program that alerts the immune system to identify this substance as a foreign invader.

Special immune system cells identify and tag this substance, and other immune system cells called phagocytes rush to the "invader" and try to digest it like miniature Pac-Man creatures.

When the body is not overloaded and responds in its normal way, the immune complexes are fully degraded and eliminated through the kidneys, urine, bowel, breath and skin.

When the body is overloaded and too many immune system complexes are not eliminated, or the body collects and confuses this substance with itself, the substance is programmed as an allergen.

With too many toxic substances, the body then overreacts with many immune mediators, swelling, inflammation and an overabundance of histamine. The brain is then programmed for an allergic overreaction. This allergy program can also be connected with a negative emotion creating or triggering the allergy response.

The allergy response begins to block electromagnetic pathways, nerve and lymph circulation, etc. This creates abnormal and destructive tissue responses and autoimmune reactions.

We use spinal/cranial adjusting techniques, percussion, the Erchonia 635 nm low-level laser, acupuncture-acupressure techniques, color and/or sound therapy, etc., to bring back balance to areas that were blocked and teach the brain and body to adopt the new corrected program.

When the person with the allergy/sensitivity holds the offending substance in the hand, just as Dr. Nambudripad held the carrot accidentally, the brain and energy field can learn a new program with the proper rewriting of the script. The brain and immune system can learn that the electromagnetic field of the allergen is not threatening. The body's new coherent energy program then neutralizes excess immune system activity and eliminates the allergic response. A process of desensitization has taken place.

178

The desensitizing process isn't always instant. It takes 24 hours for energy to fully pass through all of the body's 12 paired electromagnetic pathways or meridians. We recommend avoidance of the treated food or substance for 25 hours so that the new peaceful program will not be confused with the old aggressive program that put the immune system into overdrive.

If you have many sensitivities, it may take multiple appointments to help you on your journey to wellness. Remember, health is not a destination; it's a journey. This journey takes removing all 6 interference patterns for you to accomplish wellness fully and completely.

When all of the 6 Interferences to Health are identified and removed with the Six Steps to Wellness, the body knows how to heal itself. The body needs no help; it just needs no interference.

Only glimpses of our many techniques are discussed in this book, and are intended to inform patients and interest Wellness Practitioners, Coaches, and Doctors to learn more. Hands-on instruction is important for proficiency, and is taught by the Brimhall Wellness Team at many seminars throughout each year. For more information, please visit our website: www.brimhall.com or call our office: (866) 338-4883.

SUMMARY

- An allergy or sensitivity is the result of an abnormal immune system reaction to a substance that a healthy body treats as harmless.
- One can react to substances in the environment and food or food additives.
- Allergy/sensitivity patterns can be reprogrammed so that the body stops over-reacting to harmless substances as if they were foreign invaders.
- The A/SERT technique involves identifying the offending substances, eliminating them temporarily and reprogramming the body through the *6 Steps To Wellness*.

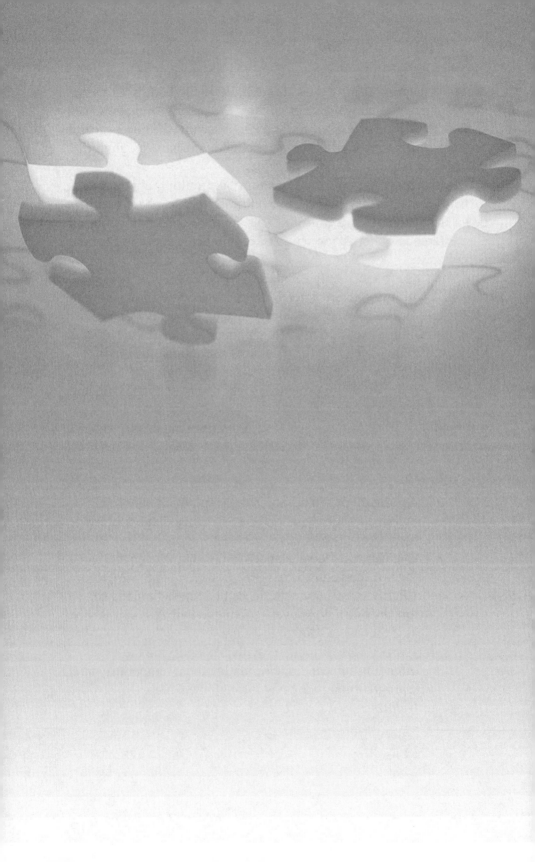

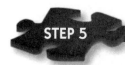

RE-EVALUATE EMOTIONAL PATTERNS AND REMOVE LIMITING BELIEF SYSTEMS

Now we move into areas of the mind and emotions. It's generally accepted now that negative thoughts can precipitate emotional and physical disorders, and positive thoughts can enhance health, and help reverse both physical and emotional problems. When unhealthy emotional patterns are removed, the normal health and vitality of the mind and body can resume.

Techniques, such as guided imagery, positive suggestion therapy, subliminal tapes, tuning forks (sound therapy), deep breathing, integration of the spine, percussion of restricted fascial patterns, cold laser and color therapy may be used individually, or in synergy, to trigger the release of negative emotional patterns and replace them with positive ones.

Guided-imagery techniques can help you use the mind-body connection to your advantage. Guided imagery uses thinking in visual images to give you positive thoughts that trigger a healthy immune response.

People who have to live with chronic pain can alleviate the burden of pain by replacing the sensation of discomfort with an imagined sensation of warmth. This technique is commonly used in biofeedback training with many variations.

Neurolinguistic programming may also help increase health. What we say to ourselves can affect our health either negatively or positively.

I THINK, THEREFORE I AM

When your language to yourself is negative, you get negative results. When your self-talk is positive, you reprogram your mind and emotions to feel and behave in positive ways. When you say you can, you do. When you say you can't, you don't. Your feelings follow your words, and your body walks in step with your language habits.

Although acupuncture is known for its beneficial effects on

pain reduction, it has also been extremely successful in removing addictions to drugs and alcohol, as well as many emotional problems including nervous disorders, worry, depression, insomnia, criminal behaviors, paranoid schizophrenia and personality disorders.

Common results of removing negative patterns include:

- Improved social interaction
- Reduced aggression
- Improved clarity of thought
- Calmer, less agitated behavior

Acupuncture techniques can be extended for swift and lasting gains by touching, tapping or lasering acupoint areas.

Color can be used to identify emotional issues as well as release them. Color therapy techniques, applied directly to the eyes with color therapy eyewear, help identify negative patterns and replace them with positive patterns. Flashing eyelights can change brain patterns.

Flower remedies have been shown to successfully balance negative feelings and stress and to help remove emotional barriers to health. The body knows how to heal itself when it's not interfered with emotionally, physically or with any of the 6 Interferences. There's no reason you must be held hostage by your feelings.

• • • • • • • • • • • • • • • • • • • •

A Case of Depression, Sleep Problems and More

I came to your clinic with the desire to get off the medications I was taking for depression, sleep problems, and migraines. Also, I had been losing my hair, was having pain during intercourse and while urinating, plus neck aches and body aches. I weaned myself off of my medications, or reduced them significantly. Other improvements include: very little to no neck pain (after 25 years of pain!), little pain in my lower back (after 35 years!), no more hair loss, a better depression level and no pain or burning in urination or intercourse. I don't ache and I can sleep better. I have been practicing imagery and pushing negative energy through an imaginary hole on the top of my head. You taught me how to make it work. I have so much energy. Thanks!

— Reneé H.

ENERGY IN MOTION

Emotion (e-motion) means energy in motion. Emotions are not the problem; but health is affected when emotions get stuck and the motion or expression of thoughts, past events or concepts are not allowed to move. Zig Zigler calls this "stinkin' thinkin." Many different authors have many different ideas about causes and treatments for stress or emotional abnormalities. In wellness care, we often take an energy-balance approach.

We have past experiences, family influences and limiting belief systems that influence our decisions and the way we relate to the world. If we want to progress and be well in all aspects of our lives, it's paramount not to spend life looking in our rear-view mirrors. We must acknowledge the past, work through it and move to the present to mold the future we desire. If it was an experience you don't want to repeat, admit it, quit it and forget it.

The body does work like a computer. All memories and events are recorded on the hard drive of the body. If you can bring up the event, memory or concept, etc., and look at it on the screen, you can erase it, just like you do on the computer. "Impossible!" you say? We know! People have been telling us what is impossible our whole lives, even after we have been able to do it over and over again.

Positive Point Therapy

The positive points are on the forehead, approximately one inch from the midline and halfway between the hairline and the eyebrows.

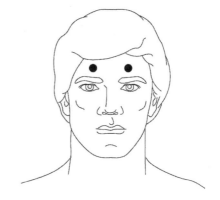

Instructions

1. Concentrate on a potentially stress-producing situation (such as a test or job interview, a memory of a divorce or an old resentment) and visualize the event of past or recent trauma or

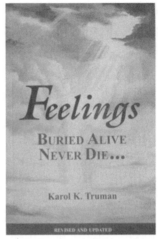

some recurrent negative pattern. Concentrate on a potentially stress-producing situation (such as a test, job interview, etc.). Visualize the concept of past or recent trauma, (accident, divorce, loss of a loved one), or recurrent negative pattern.

2. Close your eyes and allow yourself to fully experience the image and/or to experience the associated tension connected with the image.

3. While you're experiencing the image, lightly touch the point above each eye with the fingertips of each hand for approximately 10 seconds. The energy and emotion behind the event will diminish, or you will feel a release or disconnection from the force of the event.

4. Repeat steps 2 and 3 until the event no longer triggers an emotional stress response, or you feel that the stress related to the event has decreased significantly. This procedure may take 2, 3 or up to 10 repetitions to complete.

5. It's recommended that you use this technique again in potentially stressful situations (before, during or afterward) to continue to clear this kind of trauma or recurrent negative pattern. It's simple, costs nothing and is very effective.

A Case of Feelings That Were "Buried Alive"

Dear Dr. Brett,

I am so glad that I faced up to things and released the pent-up emotions at your office. This was an experience I will never forget. I feel so much better. It's helped me realize that I need to go to a whole new level of trusting God and appreciating what He does for me and the joy He gives me, even when it's something that causes me pain. For the first time ever, I can comfortably say to myself, "I'm somebody. I've got a place in this world. I'm supposed to be here. God put me here, and I'm worthy of love and a great life." That's the most precious gift I could ever receive.

— Lisa J.

SEE THE WORLD THROUGH ROSE-COLORED GLASSES

Color therapy is the use of color in assisting the body in its natural ability to balance itself. Practitioners of the healing arts have used color for centuries. Color serves to support our vital life force by supplying light energy to the system. Color can relieve stress, stimulate energy, alleviate pain and alter mood.

The body needs all electromagnetic wavelengths of natural sunlight for its circadian rhythms, including healthy sleep cycles and cycles of hormone production. Specific parts of this electromagnetic spectrum are analyzed by the eye and perceived as color. When color enters our body, it stimulates the pineal and pituitary glands, stimulating hormones and other physical processes.

Each color corresponds to a particular area of the body as well as a particular state of mind. The cooler colors have sedative, relaxing effects, while the warmer colors are warming and stimulating.

Blue lowers blood pressure, heart rate and respiration rate. Blue can make a hot room seem cooler and alleviates pain and inflammation of many kinds.

Green benefits people with depression and anxiety, alleviates nervous disorders and exhaustion and helps in dieting.

Violet suppresses appetite, alleviates migraine headaches and is good for scalp and kidney disorders.

Red helps increase confidence, stimulates brain wave activity, aids in impotence and frigidity, stimulates heart rate and is helpful for skin, bladder and anemia.

Pink soothes mind and body. It has a tranquilizing effect on aggressive and violent people and is used in hospitals, prisons, juvenile centers and drug centers.

Orange alleviates depression, weakness, allergies and fatigue and stimulates the appetite.

Yellow alleviates depression, stimulates memory and relieves cramps, hypoglycemia, overactive thyroid and gallstones.

Black is a power color, which, like red, enhances strength and self-confidence. It also helps suppress appetite.

Color Therapy Eyewear is one means of directing color energy into the body. The eyes convert electromagnetic frequencies of different parts of the spectrum into what we perceive as color. The body further converts this energy into electricity, which travels through our nervous system, directing all body functions. When a color frequency enters our eyes, each frequency is directed to the area of the body that recognizes that particular frequency. This can cause positive cellular and hormonal changes to occur, synchronizing the body with the color.

Color Therapy Eyewear lenses are non-prescription, colored sunglasses designed to make the use of color therapy convenient and affordable. Colored Glasses come in nine individual colors: red, orange, yellow, green, blue, indigo, violet, aqua and magenta. We teach the practitioners how to evaluate and treat the patients with color therapy, many times to immediate and great success.

COLORS AND CHAKRAS

The word "chakra" is found in ancient Sanskrit writings. Chakras are described as spinning focal points of energy present only in subtle matter, which directly relate to the endocrine system. Chakras exist all over the body and their function is to receive, process and transmit energy, which affects the physical, emotional and subtle energy levels of the body. We use color to balance the chakras to great advantage.

CHAKRA CHART

AQUA: corresponds to the thymus, and is a helper in working through grief. Aqua balance is a merging of heart and words to produce loving expressions.

MAGENTA: corresponds to the vitality of the system offering healing support and emotional balance.

VIOLET: corresponds to the pineal gland, cerebral cortex, right eye, central nervous system, upper brain function. Violet balance is universal love, spiritual motivation and understanding, open to divine wisdom, selfless. Violet is "I Know." Complementary color is Yellow.

INDIGO: corresponds to the pituitary gland, left eye, sinus, nose, sight. Indigo balance is inspirational, focus, concentration, insight, imagination, devotion, clear thinking, peace of mind. Indigo is "I See." Complementary color is Yellow/Orange.

BLUE: corresponds to the throat, thyroid, parathyroid, lungs, mouth. Blue balance is freedom of expression verbally and artistically, integrity, honesty, loyalty, reliability, gentleness, kindness, commitment, endurance. Blue is "I Speak." Complementary color is Orange.

GREEN: corresponds to the heart, circulatory system, arms, hands. Green balance is openness, compassion, unconditional love, forgiveness, acceptance, contentment, nurturing, generous, harmonious, assertive, heals loss. Green is "I Love." Complementary color is Red.

YELLOW: corresponds to the solar plexus, stomach, liver, gallbladder, pancreas. Yellow balance is logic, humor, efficiency, organized, warm, radiant, flexible, self aware, self-control, personal power. Yellow is "I Can." Complementary color is Violet.

ORANGE: corresponds to the reproductive organs, genitals, gonads, prostate, spleen. Orange balance is sensuality, passions, procreation, vitality, optimism, enthusiasm, hospitable, family oriented, tolerant. Orange is "I Feel." Complementary color is Blue.

RED: corresponds to the base of the spine, adrenals, kidneys, bladder, colon, spinal column, legs, blood. Red balance is in relation to the physical, self-preservation, survival, sensory, instinctual, stable, secure, primal, grounded, spontaneous, active, courageous. Red is "I Have." Complementary color is Green.

· ·

STOP AND SMELL THE ROSES

Flower remedies can help balance negative feelings and stress and remove emotional barriers to health. In 1938, an English physician, Edward Bach, developed homeopathic flower remedies to treat the emotional base of physical illness. "Treat people for their emotional unhappiness, allow them to be happy, and they will become well," Bach said.

Numerous studies at medical centers and universities have verified his conviction. The practice of flower remedy involves thinking of the patient first: focusing on what the patient's feelings and concerns are, rather than focusing on a physical disease or the symptoms of the physical disease.

Bach believed that physical disease was only symptomatic of the real cause: a negative emotional state, such as:

- Jealousy
- Fear
- Anxiety
- Insecurity
- Anger
- Poor self-image
- Shyness
- Resentment

When emotions are balanced, general health can improve and illness can dissipate. Psychoneuroimmunology studies the effects of the effects of psychological and emotional states on suppressing or stimulating the immune system, cellular activity, adrenal gland hormones and neurotransmitters.

Flower remedies are gentle, subtle, non-addictive and without side effects, and the need for their use declines over time. They are helpful when combined with acupuncture (energy or meridian balancing) and a technique we call Brain Balance. Acupuncture and Brain Balance, release blocked energy channels and negative emotional energy that has been stored. (The term acupuncture is used generically here to mean energy or meridian balancing.) Sound and music have long been recognized as having powerful effects on health. From biblical accounts of David's soothing harp to ancient Greek writings of energetic drumbeats, sound therapy and music have always been used in healing.

HEY! WHAT'S THAT HEALING SOUND?

Sound and music are used in corporations, hospitals, schools and by psychological treatment practitioners to accelerate learning, overcome learning disabilities, reduce stress, increase endurance and strength, increase cerebral and peripheral circulation and increase mental clarity.

Noise is recognized to produce nervousness and stress, though certain sounds and slow music can slow breathing and help create feelings of well-being. Music can reduce blood pressure, alter skin temperature, influence brain wave frequencies and alleviate muscle tension.

Sound, like color, is a part of a spectrum. The spectrum of sound is composed of oscillating waves of energy perceived within an audible range. Rhythmic sounds outside the body entrain the heartbeat to beat in step with the beat of drums or the pulse of the music source.

Resonance or pitch stimulates different parts of the body: lower sounds stimulate the lower parts of the body, while higher pitches stimulate higher parts of the body.

Sound is linked to the body by the eighth and tenth cranial nerves. These nerves carry sound impulses, via the skull, and ear to the frequency monitors in the brain. Motor and sensory impulses are then sent through the vagus nerve, affecting breathing rhythm, speech and heart rate.

In health, the internal rhythms among heart, breathing, organs and craniosacral systems are synchronized. In illness, the internal rhythms of breathing, heart rate, craniosacral systems and organs are disturbed. Sound and music help reset the body's rhythms so the body can heal itself.

Sound and music have helped teach people with autism, dyslexia, learning dysfunctions and attention deficit disorders to listen attentively and focus.

In the hospital and in dentistry, music is used to relax patients before, during and following surgery. Tonal music has been used effectively to enhance or replace anesthesia.

LISTEN TO YOUR BODY ... LITERALLY

Biosonic Repatterning, developed by John Beaulieu, ND, PhD, is a natural method of healing. A form of biosonic repatterning can be used to affect our nervous systems, which synchronize in much the same way as when we find a pitch for a choir or tune a piano. The vestibular system, via the semi-circular canals, can reset and rebalance the nervous system. During the listening process, our physical body will actually re-posture itself to hold the sound correctly.

John Beaulieu discovered Biosonic Repatterning while sitting in an anechoic chamber (a soundproof room resembling a sensory-deprivation chamber) at New York University. A composer-philosopher, John Cage, found that he had heard two sounds while in the chamber. One was a high-pitched sound and the other a low-pitched sound. The engineer he was working with informed him that the high sound was his nervous system, and the low sound was his blood in circulation.

Excited by this discovery, John Beaulieu then sat in an anechoic chamber for five hundred hours over a period of two years, listening to the sounds of his own body. He began to correlate different states of consciousness with the different sounds of his nervous system. Being a trained musician, he noticed that the high-pitched sounds of his nervous system consisted of several sounds in different intervals. His discoveries are now used to help realign feelings and parts of the body's structures.

To understand this process, remember a time when you were in a quiet place. During this time, you may have heard a high-pitched sound in your head. This is the sound of your nervous system. When you're under stress, this sound gets louder and sometimes can become a ringing in the ears. For most of us, this sound is subtle, and we only hear it when we focus on it.

Tuning into the sound of your nervous system is a kind of meditation. Find a quiet place, sit or lie down, close your eyes and focus your awareness on the sounds inside your head. Listen for the high sound. When you listen closely, you'll discover that the sound consists of two distinct pitches. These pitches originate from your left and right brain hemispheres. These pitches change in frequency, volume and pitch depending on your state of consciousness.

As you listen to the two different tones, your body will naturally adjust itself and come into balance, making the two sounds into one. You can hum and let your voice resonate with the sound of the interval. This humming creates a sonic anchor, which helps you rebalance your feelings and body.

Some Correlations Among Sound, Colors, Music and Toning

Color	Note	Scale	Music Instrument
Violet	B	Ti	Transcendental Winds
Indigo	A	La	Classical Reeds
Blue	G	So	Country/Western Fine Strings
Green	F	Fa	Easy Listening Piano
Yellow	E	Mi	Structural Jazz Harp
Orange	D	Re	Folk, Reggae Thick Strings
Red	C	Do	Rock 'n' Roll Bass Tones

GET BACK TO THE WOMB

We frequently use guided-imagery sessions in conjunction with other modalities, such as color therapy, verbal affirmations and structural corrections, to replace negative patterns. These techniques can result in powerful releases and changes in one's life and health.

During a guided-imagery session, the subject lays face up on the table. The practitioner may hold the patient's cranium and perform a craniosacral release, use the Erchonia 635 nm low-level laser, or use an appropriate tuning fork over key energy points on the body. The practitioner can also use his or her hands, percussor, or cold laser on the structural area that needs release.

It is important that you are not interrupted during this process. Be aware that the subject may cry or otherwise release emotions. Emotional release should be expected as normal and good. This is encouraged and supported, as great healing takes place here. The practitioner or tableside assistant will verbally guide the patient's mental imagery. The patient may or may not respond verbally.

The following is an example of a guided-imagery script:
"Close your eyes and think about what was going on in your life when your health problem started. Get in touch with that time of your life. Feel your emotions. What was your state of mind? What were your surroundings like? What are the specific emotions? Try to see them as tangible. What color are they? Size? Shape? Do they have a smell? Taste?"

(The practitioner should speak in calm, soft tones and pause from time to time, allowing the patient to think about the words.)

"FIVE-MINUTE PHOBIA CURE"

Psychologist Roger Callahan developed a concept called the "Five-Minute Phobia Cure." He found that popular scriptures speak the truth. To love your neighbor as yourself means you must first love yourself. People have to forgive themselves of their weakness before they can overcome it.

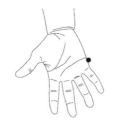

Callahan found that kinesiology could be used to aid in this process. A computer speaks in a binary language (one's or zeroe's, or yese's and noe's). The body also speaks in this binary language and can be monitored with yes and no answers with muscle response testing.

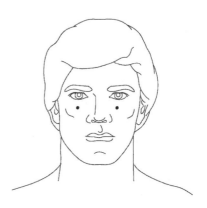

The best way to see the impact of this technique is to do it. First, identify the fear, phobia or habit to overcome. Verbally declare, "I totally and completely love myself even though I have ___ problem" (fear, phobia, habit, etc.) If a previously strong muscle goes weak after making this statement, then tap the acupuncture point SI 3 (small intestine 3) with both hands together. This point is identified by making a fist with both hands, with the palm sides facing you. Tap the outsides of the hands (between the pinkies and heels of the hands) together while you verbally declare, "I totally and completely love myself, even though ___," three times.

The second part to this technique is done by the person rating the problem, fear, phobia or habit, on a scale from one to ten, according to perceived severity. The person then visualizes this number decrease in their mind, while tapping acupuncture points St 1½ (Stomach 1½), at each side of the nose. The severity rating diminishes because this trapped energy is being released. You don't have to try to make it go down, it does so on its own. The person undergoing this technique will then stay strong with muscle testing.

On occasion, the number will go part way down and stop. Dr. Callahan calls this, "self-sabotage" which occurs when one doubts him/herself, or the technique. To correct this, begin again by tapping the outside hand creases (SI 3) again and saying, "I totally and completely love myself even though ___," three more times. If you have a tendency to be very negative, or this is a highly negative situation, it may take several times to get the numbers to drop consistently. They may drop one at a time or several at once.

"I totally and completely love and forgive myself, although I am afraid of spiders," which is repeated three times while the creases (SI 3) of both hands are tapped together. Then, if the numerical rating of the fear of spiders is a ten, the patient taps at the side of their nose, while visualizing the number drop from ten, six, three... one, zero.) The patient will not be afraid of spiders anymore. We have found this technique to be about 90% effective.

You say it can't be that easy? Remember, the body functions as a holographic bio-computer, so think in computer terms. You boot up the computer, pull the file you want to work on up onto the screen. If you don't like what it says, simply highlight it and push delete. Then, rewrite a script the way you want it to read. That is the same way the body works. Yes, it does seem like a miracle to.................
experience it. Isn't that the point, though, that life and the body are miracles? An example of this technique: We once treated a lovely lady in her sixties who came to us after she had lost her husband to a serious illness. She had spent hundreds of thousands of dollars on

medical bills and had become ill, herself, from stress, to the point that she could no longer drive. She would experience panic attacks, freeze in the middle of an intersection and just sit in her car and cry. We had her do both parts of this technique. She declared, three times, that she totally and completely loved herself, even though she was afraid to drive, while tapping the creases of her hands. She then rated the fear and tapped the sides of her nose until the number decreased to zero. Afterward, she felt better, but was still unsure she could operate a car when alone.

We then had her process, "I love myself even though I'm afraid to be alone," and then rate and tap until that number fell to zero. She also processed through both steps with the fear of financial disaster and several other related feelings. There were multiple issues, so we just processed them one at a time. The end result was wellness, driving again and eventually meeting and marrying a very nice gentleman.

Did this woman live happily ever after and have no more problems in life? Yes and no. She is still alive today, is able to drive again and is enjoying her life and family. But, if she expected a life with no problems, she came to the wrong planet. That is why we are teaching her (and you) the things to help the journey.

Our understanding is that we came to this earth to experience challenges and grow from them. That's why we keep saying, "Wellness is a journey and not a destination." We must learn the rules of a joyous life and seek God's guidance in His plan for us.

SUMMARY

- Negative thoughts can precipitate emotional and physical disorders.
- Positive thoughts enhance health and reverse both physical and emotional problems..
- Guided imagery can reduce stress, slow the heart rate and stimulate the immune system.
- What we say to ourselves, our internal dialogue, affects our health, either negatively or positively.
- Acupressure techniques release negative emotional patterns and replace them with positive patterns.
- Acupressure, guided imagery, Brain Balance,

subliminal tapes, structural techniques, color therapy, sound therapy and flower remedies allow emotional blocks to surface and release.

- The body knows how to heal itself, when it is not interfered with by limiting belief systems or any of the 6 Interferences to Health.

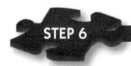

REMOVE HEAVY METALS AND OTHER TOXINS FROM THE BODY

Toxins are everywhere, many of them have a heavy metal base. Several years ago, they removed lead from gasoline and from paint. We hear on the news, very often, about the controversy of having mercury in vaccinations. Some say, it can cause autism. Asbestos was found to cause cancer; wherever they find asbestos they remove it. Later in this chapter, we have listed a few of the individual heavy metals and some of the problems they can cause. Years back, there were the "No-pest Strips." The convenience to hang them around to ward off bugs was great; but, it created other not-so-convenient problems.

The EPA estimates that the users of "No-pest strips" face a cancer risk much greater than those who never used it. Flea collars with the same dichlorvos (2.2-dichlorvinyl dimethyl phosphate or DVVP) put animals at a similar risk.

Lead acetate is the leading ingredient in many over-the-counter hair dyes. A study by Xavier University in New Orleans by an associate professor of toxicology said these dyes, when used as directed, spread lead acetate from the hands to whatever they touch.

The associate professor believes they should be taken off the shelves and that the greatest threat is to children and pregnant women. According to the study, the dyes themselves contain up to 5,954 mcg of lead per gram, far above the 600 mcg/g allowed in paint.

GOT DRUGS?

In 1989, studies were conducted on samples of low-fat and skim milk from grocery shelves. In one case 38% were found to be contaminated with sulfa drugs or antibiotics. In another case, 20% were similarly contaminated.

IT'S NOT A GAS

In March of 2000, the EPA announced plans to phase down, and possibly eliminate the use of the suspected carcinogen MTBE, an octane booster used in gasoline. The chemical, which reduces a vehicle's emissions, "now taints drinking-water supplies throughout the nation," according to an article in *Science News*.

Much of the U.S. contamination threatens groundwater. Underground fuel tanks, many beneath gas stations, are a primary source; some 250,000 of them leak MTBE-laced gasoline.

ENVIRONMENTAL ILLNESS AND WOMEN

Women may be more susceptible to pollutants, than men, because they have more body fat. Toxins are stored in fat and pregnancy, breastfeeding, dieting, menopause and aging can all release fat, therefore releasing toxins.

SUBTRACT THOSE ADDITIVES!

In a letter to the editor, Ian D. Murphy, MD, noted that he saw no Type II Diabetes in young people when he first started practice in the early 1960's; however, it was not uncommon by 1995. Murphy believes Monosodium Glutamate (MSG) played a role. When it's fed to baby rats for their first nine days of life, it destroys the arcuate nucleus of the pituitary gland, and for the rest of their lives they're obese, hypothyroid and lethargic.

THALLIUM

One of the lesser-known heavy metals, Thallium, can be consumed by eating contaminated fruits and vegetables (all the more reason to eat organic!) or tobacco products.

The soil gets contaminated by atmospheric Thallium from coal-fired plants, smelting and cement factories. Sleep disorders, weakness, nervousness, headache and other neurological and muscular symptoms were reported in people consuming fruits and vegetables near a cement plant in Germany.

PERCHLORATE

Perchlorate is a toxic, thyroid hormone-disrupting salt that has been discovered in common household fertilizers. In September of 1999, the EPA added perchlorate to its list of contaminants that water utilities must monitor.

IN YOUR OWN BACKYARD

Backyard trash burning was found to be a major source of dioxins spewing into the environment. Researchers figured out that 2-3 people burning 1.5 kg of trash, on any given day, could match the daily dioxin output of a well-run municipal incinerator serving the needs of up to 120,000 households.

WHAT A WASTE

The *Rocky Mountain News* carried a 2001 story headlined "Plutonium Confirmed at Lowry." Cleanup officials at Lowry Landfill acknowledged low levels of plutonium and other manmade radioactive contaminants in the site's groundwater.

WATCH WHAT YOU DRINK!

A report from the National Research Council in Washington, DC, suggested that drinking-water regulations need revising. Major utilities release much wastewater effluent into drinking-water supplies. The report notes, "regulators scout for less than the full spectrum of toxicants now present in that water."

THE PROBLEM AND SOME SOLUTIONS

In a 300-page report from a study done in 1979, The US Environmental Protection Agency reported that toxic metals are the second-worst environmental health problem in the United States. Toxic metals are widely used in industry, food processing and agriculture, and find their way into our air, food and water.

Good habits that can change your intake and uptake of toxic metals include eating organic, whole foods and maintaining a high-fiber diet. You must avoid conventional foods grown with pesticides and artificial fertilizers. Stay out of the canned-foods aisles. Canned and processed foods are stripped of the good nutrients and micronutrients that protect us from heavy-metal poisoning.

If your supermarket carries a fresh organic foods section, spend your time there. If the meat department has a selection of natural meats from animals raised without antibiotics and artificial hormones, that's the place you go for meat protein. If not, make the health food store your choice, and select a wide variety of fresh fruits and vegetables, and natural, unpolluted meats and fish.

"The essential trace elements are much more important than the vitamins," wrote Henry A. Schroeder, MD, in *The Poisons Around Us, Toxic Metals in Food, Air, and Water*. Essential trace elements are 50 to 800% more abundant in whole organic foods than in conventionally raised foods. Macronutrients, sulfur-based proteins, fatty acids and carbohydrates can be up to eight times more abundant.

Organic foods will cost you more money, but they'll help save your health by avoiding the pollutants and providing your body with the protective nutrition it deserves.

Choose high-sulfur foods such as onions, garlic, legumes and eggs to assist your body in blocking uptake and removing retention of many toxic metals. Choose free-range organic eggs, which have the same beneficial essential fatty acids as wild ocean-run fish, without the potential of mercury pollution.

Use only stainless steel, glass, enameled, or iron cookware, and certainly avoid aluminum cookware to reduce your intake of harmful metals.

Read labels and avoid products known to contain toxic metals. Avoid:
- Canned foods (any food in aluminum, tin, or lead-soldered cans)
- Canned beverages (soda, beer, etc.)

Peel down the label on most tomato sauces, and you will see the lead seam. Some researchers estimate we could easily reduce our lead intake 50% by simply avoiding lead-seamed canned foods.

Consider the mercury amalgam or "silver" fillings some dentists still put in your mouth. Many feel it much safer to use biologically compatible fillings. Be very selective of a Biological Dentist in removal of amalgam fillings. If a dentist isn't trained in safe removal, the filling removal itself can place more mercury in your system and make matters worse.

Include organic apples in your diet as a source of pectin, which binds with and helps remove most toxic metals from the body. Eat buckwheat, high in rutin, a protective agent against heavy metals and radiation.

FOOT BATH DETOXIFICATION

Our clinic staff is trained in the use of cold laser treatment and can help you facilitate detoxification, by increasing blood and lymph circulation. This helps remove toxins of all kinds from your tissues. We also use a unit called the EB305 (energy balancer) or the EBPRO that uses water as a medium for detoxification. We have found these machines very effective in detoxification, and because detoxifying our bodies is so important, we use them in our offices and homes.

The EB305 and EBPRO are both manufactured by Erchonia and are being researched to determine what toxins are being eliminated from the water.

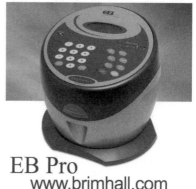

Footbath treatments are done by placing the patient's feet in a container of water with the instrument array. Specific, ionic frequencies pass through the water, and help balance the body energies and helps release toxins through pores in the feet. The water becomes discolored as toxins accumulate. This treatment lasts approximately 20-30 minutes.

EB Pro
www.brimhall.com

The patient often continues to release toxins for several days after completing a footbath. To maximize effectiveness, we recommend the patient increase their fluid intake and take other nutritional support, such as essential fatty acids, vegetable green drinks, and other specific nutrients the patient may test for.

Call Brimhall Wellness at 866-338-4883 for Certified Brimhall Practitioners or ordering of any of the products or services mentioned in this book. Also visit www.brimhall.com.

- - - - - - - - - - - - - - - - - - -

SELF-DETOXIFYING BATHS:

Epsom Salts and Ginger Bath: This bath works well to relieve the aches that accompany the flu or exercise. It opens pores and eliminates toxins. Boil freshly sliced or grated ginger root, and then let steep for 10 minutes. Mix ginger water with one cup of Epsom salts and add to a tub of water.

Salt and Soda Bath: This bath counteracts the effects of radiation from x-rays, cancer treatment, atmosphere fallout, and/or television and computer screens. It is also good for general detoxification. Add one cup of baking soda and 1-2 cups of Epsom salt to a tub of water.

Vinegar Bath: This is excellent for excess uric acid in the body and for joint problems: arthritis, bursitis, tendonitis, gout, and heavy-metal toxicity. It is a quick way to restore acid-alkaline balance. Add 1 cup to 2 quarts of 100 % apple cider vinegar to a bathtub of warm water. Find real apple cider vinegar in a health foods store. (Most "apple cider" vinegars are flavored grain vinegars, as indicated by the bottle's labeling.)

COFFEE ENEMAS

Although coffee may not be a suitable beverage for you, it's a very effective agent for cleansing the liver when used as an enema. There may be no better stimulant for bile production and its subsequent flushing, than coffee. This is due to a number of pharmacologically acting substances in the coffee. The combination of theobromine, theophylline and caffeine in coffee stimulates the relaxation of smooth muscles, causing dilation of blood vessels and bile ducts.

Hence, bile flow is increased.

The coffee enema is unsurpassed in its capacity to stimulate the flushing of toxic bile, or bile that has been loaded with toxins by the glutathione-S-transferase system. It has literally been a lifesaver to many hundreds of people undergoing extreme detoxification.

The use of enemas, in certain cases, proves to be very beneficial in the detoxification process and has enabled patients to progress at a faster rate than they would normally have been able to.

The effects of taking a coffee enema are not the same as drinking coffee. The coffee enema is absorbed into the hemorrhoid vein, and then taken up by the portal vein, which serves the liver directly. The enema is retained for 15 minutes, during which time it stimulates the liver cells to cleanse the blood, removing toxins. The liver's entire blood circulation will be recycled about five times during this period, enabling a thorough cleanse.

With the bile ducts open, a flushing of toxic bile is encouraged, which enters the gastro-intestinal tract. The large volume of fluid retained in the lower colon stimulates peristaltic activity, which ensures the propulsion of bile through the intestine to the outside. It's important to remember that the enema is given for the stimulation of the liver and not for the function of the intestines.

A coffee-retention enema is quite helpful during a serious illness, after hospitalization and after exposure to toxic chemicals. This enema can also be used during fasts to relieve the headaches sometimes caused by a fast-induced release of toxins.

Take three tablespoons of <u>organic</u> ground coffee (don't use instant) and add one pint of water. The pollutant chemicals found in commercially grown coffee could damage the liver when used as a coffee enema, so use only organically grown coffee! Bring the water to a boil for three minutes, and then allow the solution to simmer for another 15 minutes. Strain this solution and dilute with up to one pint of water. When the solution has reached body temperature (when it's comfortable to put your elbow into the solution), pour this into an enema bag.

Take this solution into the bowel as an enema and retain as long as possible. Change positions while retaining the coffee. After a few minutes, turn over onto your back. A few minutes later switch to your left side before evacuating your bowels.

Cautions: Two coffee enemas in a week, during a cleansing

period, are good for most people, but not for everyone. If coffee enemas make you feel worse, even when using organic coffee, you should discontinue using them.

WHICH METALS ARE HURTING YOU?

Sometimes we recommend taking homeopathic remedies for body balance and toxic-metal contamination. We also use a nutrient combination called Total Chelate™ to assist in detoxification. Of course nutritional support for liver detoxification is also an important consideration.

Hair analysis, blood studies and other lab tests can be helpful in testing for body burden of heavy metals and other toxins.

HOMEOPATHIC REMEDIES

Homeopathic remedies are one non-toxic solution to body and health balance. Homeopathic remedies are based on the reverse conception, "If a little is good, a lot is better." In other words if onions make you cry, diluted onion juice will stop tearing in many people if you get the right dilution. The science is finding out the right remedy and the right dilution of that remedy.

In homeopathy, the more a substance is diluted, the higher the potency of its effects. The Law of the Infinitesimal Dose was discovered by Dr. Hahnemann by experimentation with higher and higher dilutions to avoid toxic side effects.

Homeopathic remedies are diluted in water or alcohol to such an extent that no molecules of the original substance remain. Any homeopathic remedy over 24X potency (24 successive dilutions and succussions) contains no molecular trace of the original substance. However, an imprint of the original substance does remain.

A study using Nuclear Magnetic Resonance (NMR) imaging demonstrated readings of distinguishing subatomic activity in 23 different homeopathic remedies tested, but this distinguishing activity was not present in placebos.

Some homeopathic researchers believe that the specific electromagnetic frequency of the original substance is imprinted on the homeopathic remedy by successive dilution. This theory was given credibility by a German biophysicist, Wolfgang Ludwig, who demonstrated that diluted homeopathic substances do give off measurable electromagnetic signals. Mae-Wan Ho's understanding of biophysics further supports this: hydrogen-based liquid crystalline structures learn, have memories, and can act as messengers.

"Dr. Richard Gerber explained that a homeopathic remedy conveys an electromagnetic "message," to the body, that matches the specific electromagnetic frequencies of an illness. It also stimulates the body's natural healing response." The cold laser, using frequency modulation, is thought to trigger much of the same reaction.

TOXIC METAL CONTAMINATION

We are going to just list a few of the many contaminants that are around and in us:

Mercury

Mercury amalgam or "silver" fillings are a major source of mercury exposure. Amalgams are composed of 50% mercury, 25% silver, and 25% other metals such as copper, tin and nickel, according to the World Health Organization. A single amalgam filling can release 3-17 mcg of mercury each day. Mercury vapor is released in the mouth and combines with other chemicals there to form methyl mercury, which is absorbed through mouth tissues and air passages and transported into the blood and the brain. Dentists and dental technicians who handle mercury are at greater risk because of greater daily exposures through their hands and the air.

Large fish like, yellow-fin and big-eye tuna, accumulate more mercury than smaller tuna, such as albacore. Algae, which are consumed by small fish, consume mercury-containing bacteria. Bigger fish eat the small fish, only to be eaten by humans after the mercury concentration is thousands of times greater. Fish do protect themselves, as people can protect themselves, by taking in more selenium; selenium combines with mercury to form mercury selenide, which is harmlessly excreted.

Mercury is also found in everyday products such as cosmetics, fabric softeners, inks used by tattooists and printers, latex, some medications, some paints, plastics, polishes, solvents and wood preservatives, explosives, gunpowder and some vaccinations.

Mercury pollution comes from mercury vapor lamps, batteries

and the burning of 3,000 metric tons of coal each year. Industrial workers exposed to the manufacturing of thermometers, mercury arc rectifiers, scientific equipment, or the cleaning and packing of mercury compounds, are at higher risk of poisoning.

Early toxic accumulation symptoms include: behavioral changes, depression, irritability, hyperactivity, asthma, allergies, a metallic taste in the mouth, and possible loose teeth. Significant amounts of mercury in the body can eventually produce excessive salivation, dermatitis, arthritis, gum disease, hair loss, insomnia, memory loss and muscle weakness. Mercury poisoning can mimic Lou Gehrig's Disease (ALS) and Multiple Sclerosis (MS), and it may play an important role in triggering Alzheimer's Disease, since mercury collects in the central nervous system and brain.

Negative nutritional factors: Selenium deficiency encourages absorption and retention of mercury. Most dietary mercury is found in the fat of fish. Broiling fish and draining the fatty juices will reduce intake, but retain beneficial alkyl glycerols in the meat of the fish, which help remove mercury. High-fiber, organic whole foods and high-sulfur foods reduce absorption. Supplemental zinc and Vitamin C may also help eliminate mercury poisoning. However, supplemental selenium, taken after mercury exposure, does not help eliminate mercury.

Nickel

Trace amounts of nickel are essential to humans, although its exact mechanisms are not well understood. Nickel plays a role in DNA and RNA synthesis, activates trypsin and arginase enzymes, and may play beneficial roles in membrane, hormone and lipid metabolism. Nickel deficiencies aren not believed to exist, since nickel is ubiquitous in plants, animals and in the air.

Excess nickel accumulation can cause skin rash and irritation, respiratory illness, interfere with the Kreb's energy cycle and may contribute to heart attacks. Industrial inhalation of nickel carbonyl has been linked to nasal and lung cancers, worsened by heavy tobacco smoking. Excess nickel may supersensitize the inflammatory response. Sources of nickel exposure include cocoa, chocolate, water, dental materials, hydrogenated oils and fats, processed and refined foods, buckwheat, oats, legumes, cabbage, and nickel-cadmium batteries.

Negative nutritional and lifestyle factors: Excess nickel intake can be avoided by not consuming refined and processed foods, hydrogenated fats and oils, and not using stainless-steel cookware in preparing acidic foods such as tomato sauce (use glass cookware instead). Avoid using other metal cooking utensils, and use plastic or wooden utensils instead, wood being the better of the two choices. Avoid superphosphate fertilizers and tobacco smoke. Using gold earrings and other non-nickel, plated jewelry can prevent allergic reactions to nickel in watchbands, zippers, bra closures, pierced earrings and other everyday items that come in contact with skin.

Thallium

The heavy metal thallium is found in concentrations of 0.7 ppm in the Earth's crust and is released into the atmosphere from coal-fired plants, smelting and cement factories. Thallium can be inhaled from the air and contaminate surface water and soil. No known metabolic functions have been described.

The most common sources of exposure are through consumption of fruits and vegetables grown in contaminated soil and the use of tobacco products. Before 1972, thallium was used as a rodent poison, but has since been banned because of extreme toxicity. Currently, it's used in photoelectric cells, nickel-cadmium batteries, lamps, electronics, semiconductors, organic catalysts, and in imaging procedures for myocardial disease. Uptake of thallium can be through ingestion, inhalation or dermal contact.

Thallium accumulates within the nervous system, reproductive organs, kidney, muscle, skin and brain. It inactivates riboflavin, disrupts potassium homeostasis and inhibits cholinesterase, phosphatase and RNA/DNA synthesis.

Toxic accumulation symptoms: Acute toxicity produces parathesia, neuritis, ataxia, delirium, tremors and hallucinations. Chronic exposures result in brain, spinal cord, and peripheral nerve damage. The most common indicator of long-term thallium poisoning is male-pattern baldness. Other symptoms involve anorexia, mental confusion, hypertension, and immune-function changes. Sleep disorders, weakness, nervousness, headache and other neurological and muscular symptoms were reported in people consuming fruits and vegetables near a cement plant in Germany.

As mentioned, these are just a few that could be considered. We teach doctors and practitioners that attend Brimhall Wellness Seminars, how to test for and identify over fifteen different toxic metal contaminants in their patients.

Calcium and Other Minerals to Protect Against Heavy Metals

Positive nutritional factors: Calcium, magnesium, and other minerals in adequate or large amounts, help prevent uptake and retention of radioactive metals. Taking adequate calcium, magnesium, Vitamin C, and the B Vitamins help bind with aluminum and help remove it from the colon, through the urine or the skin.

Deficiencies of calcium, copper and protein increase cadmium absorption. Zinc can give some protection against cadmium by blocking its absorption and helping remove it. Calcium and Vitamin D can reverse or prevent cadmium-caused bone softening. Copper competes with cadmium for absorption, iron protects against cadmium intake, and selenium protects against cadmium-caused tumors of testicles and cancers of connective tissue. Vitamin C and protein can protect against cadmium.

Total Calcium™ (veg): Synergistic Calcium Formula

We frequently use Total Calcium™, a synergistic blend of calcium, zinc, Vitamin C, and other healthy nutrients, to reduce excessive copper absorption. Deficiencies in calcium and other beneficial minerals increase absorption of toxic lead. High dietary calcium, magnesium and phosphorous reduce lead absorption. Elimination of lead storage in the body requires high calcium and phosphorous levels. Strengthening the activities of the eliminative organs of the skin, liver, kidney and bowel can help remove many metal poisons.

Total Calcium™ contains calcium, calcium hydroxyapatite, magnesium, manganese, parotid, zinc, copper, Vitamin D and boron with synergistic nutrients.

Boron and Synergistic Nutrients to Remove Heavy Metals

Our clinical experience and, follow-up assessments, found

that boron, in combination with other helpful nutrients, plays an important role in neutralizing the toxicities of several heavy metals. This finding may be the first report of such a beneficial role for boron.

We believe the following line of thinking may partially explain a new role for boron as a protective nutrient. First, boron has been considered a catalytic trace element in humans, plants and animals. Some of boron's roles have been identified. Albrecht, and others, have shown boron's role in liver glycogen synthesis. Bersin demonstrated that boron deficiency triggered eczema, acne and enteritis in people prone to skin allergies. Russian research suggests that boron plays a role in adrenaline, carbohydrate and fat metabolism. In chick studies, boron was first discovered to influence the metabolism of calcium, magnesium, phosphorous and Vitamin D. Boron supplementation was shown to alleviate magnesium deficiency signs in chicks.

It's this identified role, involving mineral interaction, that leads us to believe that boron plays a regulatory role in enhancing and normalizing at least three minerals that may have primary effects on protecting the body against heavy metals. By enhancing the levels of beneficial minerals known to affect heavy-metal poisoning, boron may play a regulatory role in helping the body block uptake of heavy metals and help discard them.

Deficiencies in calcium, potassium, iodine and other minerals result in an increased uptake of poisonous radioactive elements. Increased nutrient levels are known to be beneficial and help the body eliminate these elements. For example, calcium and magnesium bind with aluminum and help remove it from the body.

We theorize that boron may play a role by enhancing the levels of zinc, just as it is known to enhance the levels of other minerals.

If boron also enhances not only zinc, but also molybdenum, this regulatory enhancement would also explain improvements in copper, lead, cadmium and mercury toxicity levels.

Molybdenum alone is known to block and remove excess copper, lead, cadmium and mercury poisoning in animal studies.

In lead poisoning, deficiency in calcium and other minerals is known to increase absorption of lead. Boron is known to raise levels of calcium in calcium-deficient animals, and markedly reduce the excretion of calcium in women between 48-82 years of age. Boron also increases estrogen and testosterone levels.

We believe that boron, by enhancing the levels of hormones and beneficial minerals known to reduce heavy-metal poisoning, may play an important regulatory role in helping the body block uptake of heavy metals and help discard them. Boron is combined with steel in nuclear utility plants to trap radiation. It's also used in experimental drugs for trapping neutrons in radiation therapy, and we believe it may play a protective role against uranium, radium and radon's damaging effects.

We theorize that boron may also play a beneficial role in helping trap radiation poisoning from uranium, radium and radon, in the body, when supplemented or taken in through the diet. Boron, with synergistic nutrients, are thought to help reduce uptake of heavy metals, remove many toxic metals from the brain and intestinal tract, and help excrete heavy metal toxins from the body.

Total Boron™ (veg): For Protection Against Heavy Metals

We use a synergistic balanced nutrition, containing boron, to enhance the uptake and spare the loss of calcium, magnesium and phosphorous from the body. Both calcium and magnesium bind with aluminum, cadmium and excess copper, and help eliminate it. Adequate calcium prevents lead from being deposited in body tissues.

Calcium and magnesium help protect against radiation, especially radioactive strontium. In studies with postmenopausal women, 3 mg of boron per day significantly reduced calcium lost in the urine. Boron supplementation, in both animals and humans, results in higher estradiol, natural human estrogen levels, higher testosterone levels and higher Vitamin D levels. Low levels of boron in tissues have also been linked to lower hormonal levels. Boron is now suspected of being a mineral regulator of many minerals.

TOTAL SYSTEMIC DETOXIFICATION

We use an efficient detox supplement that addresses all seven detox pathways in the body - liver, bowel, blood, lungs, lymph, skin and kidney. All of these pathways should be detoxed, and the proper nutrients should be provided, to ensure a slow, efficient, healthy removal of stored toxins, both environmental and internal.

Total Systemic D-Tox™ (veg): Multi-vitamin/mineral/nutrient Support for Detoxification

This product contains chelators that are organic acids that bind heavy metals, antioxidants and nutrients and facilitate detox pathways. Multi-vitamin/mineral support provides energy and balance, when caloric intake has decreased, to rest the liver and optimize detox functioning. This product contains Siberian ginseng, glutathione, taurine, glycine, methionine, Vitamin C, Vitamin E, beta carotene, quercetin, selenium, coenzyme Q 10, curcurmin, zinc, N-acetyl cysteine, red beets, chlorophyll, dandelion, asparagus, broccoli, mullein and yellow dock.

DETOXIFYING THE BODY AND ARTERIES

Stresses from many sources, including toxic metals, toxins from infectious diseases, pesticides, smoking and diet, contribute to the free radicals and toxins that oxidize cholesterol, damage blood vessels and lead to age-related conditions, such as cardiovascular disease.

Cardiovascular disease (CVD) is the leading cause of death for people over 50. About 58 million Americans live with some form of CVD. What the public hasn't fully realized, is that CVD is a systemic condition, affecting not only the coronary arteries, but also the lungs, brain, kidneys and legs. Even though CVD causes over 40% of all deaths in the U.S., CVD is believed to be one of the most preventable of chronic conditions. Oral chelation is one of the best answers to this kind of toxic buildup.

• •

Nutrient Support for Oral Chelation

Total Chelate™ (Veg) is a synergistic formula for oral chelation and removal of toxic buildup. In addition to EDTA, Total Chelate™ contains Vitamin B6, Vitamin B3, niacinamide, biotin, magnesium, zinc, selenium, inositol choline, betaine HCL, sitosterol, vegetable lipase, DL methionine, apple pectin and red algae (carrageenan).

• •

WHAT IS FIBROMYALGIA?

"Fibro" refers to fibrous connective tissue that cushions the joints, "myo" refers to the muscle, and "algia" refers to pain. The term fibromyalgia (FM) usually encompasses a description of muscle and joint pain that persists for no discernible reason. It is a syndrome characterized by widespread musculoskeletal pain, and the presence of tenderness or pain in 11 or more of 18 specific points on the body. It can include tenderness, fatigue and stiffness with loss of sleep, depression and shortness of breath.

The condition has also been called fibrositis, myofascial pain, myofascial pain syndrome, psychogenic rheumatism, fibromyositis, myofascitis, tension myalgia, psychological muscle disorder and muscular fatigue syndrome. 70% of fibromyalgia patients meet diagnostic criteria for Chronic Fatigue Syndrome (CFS). The biggest difference is that the main diagnostic criterion for CFS is fatigue, whereas the main diagnostic criterion for FM is musculoskeletal pain.

THE MYSTERY DISEASE

Dr. Lynn Toohey has concluded, in her research, that the only way to really treat Fibromyalgia is by evaluating all of the Six Interferences to Health and applying the Six Steps to Wellness, discussed throughout this book, for correction.

FM has been vaguely described by some in the past as, "a clinical entity of unknown etiology." That does not say much about pinpointing causes for the syndrome. One of the theories of fibromyalgia is that a toxic overload pushes people over the edge. When the liver, and other detox organs, can't keep up with removal, these toxins deposit in muscle fibers and connective tissue, causing pain and discomfort. Toxin accumulation, of course, is the 6th of the 6 Steps to Wellness.

Many people are not aware of the sources of their toxins until insidious exposures are considered. A handful of backyard trash-burning fires, for example, can spew as much dioxin as a municipal incinerator. Remodeling a house releases more lead, from the dust, than chewing on paint chips. A letter to the editor in the *British Medical Journal* warns of future increased allergies to tomatoes, because latex has been genetically engineering into them. Just think of the toxins we are exposed to every day, in the air we breathe and the water we drink or clean with. The amount of chlorine absorbed by your body in a, 10-minute shower, equals about two gallons of tap-water consumption.

We are being exposed to more and more toxins in our everyday environment, while nutritional status, (Step 3, one of our best defenses for clearance) is declining. Fibromyalgia is just one of the chronic and stubborn syndromes that we see increasing in rapid numbers.

A daily detox program is something to be considered.

SLEEP IS CRITICAL

Deep sleep is vital for system recovery, muscle repair, and antibody production. The immune system can become hyperactive from lack of sleep alone. Step 3 and nutritional considerations can help to solve these issues as well.

Caffeine and sugar can cause sleep disturbances, while regular aerobic exercise can help facilitate good sleep patterns. Lack of serotonin can cause sleep problems. Many drugs can potentially cause FM symptoms. In fact, the drug "fenclonene" blocks the enzyme that converts tryptophan to 5-HTP, which ultimately blocks serotonin production, and can cause severe symptoms of FM.

One theory is that there is a virus attacking the HPA axis and limbic system, causing FM. (The HPA axis involves the hypothalamus, which regulates temperature, blood pressure, pulse rate, perspiration, fluid balance and other functions of the autonomic nervous system. The limbic system is associated with memory and emotion.) The other theory states that dysfunction is the physical result of long-term mental stress, and that a repeated signal over the same nerve path will eventually alter that nerve path.

• • • • • • • • • • • • • • • • • • • •

Signs and Symptoms of Fibromyalgia
- Severe fatigue (90%)
- Stiff and aching muscles
- Sleep problems
- Skin tenderness

- Pain following physical exertion
- Burning or throbbing pain
- Pain in four quadrants of body for at least three months (right and left above and below the waist)
- Joint swelling
- The pain is located in the hips, shoulder, back and neck
- Migraine or tension headaches (50%)
- TMJ problems (25%)
- Heart palpitations and chest pain
- Anxiety or depression
- Dizziness
- Memory problems – "brain fog"
- PMS and menstrual cramps
- Cold intolerance
- Dryness of the eyes and mouth
- Unexplained bruising
- Fluid retention
- Irritable bowel syndrome
- Bladder problems
- Shortness of breath

Diagram of Tender Points:
- A - base of skull beside spinal column
- B - base of back of neck
- C - top, back part of shoulder
- D - breast bone
- E - outer edge of forearm; inch below elbow
- F - shoulder blade
- G - top of hip
- H - outside of hip (upper outer quadrant of buttock)
- I - fat pad over the knee

PROBLEMS IN DEFINING CAUSES FOR FM

Leaky Gut: As early as 1913, the *British Medical Journal* reported that one of the causes for this persistent syndrome could be the, "absorption of irritating toxins from the gut" (translated to modern terms – Leaky Gut!) We use Total Leaky Gut™ nutrition to high success.

Hypothyroidism: Many people with FM have a low function of the thyroid gland, and hypothyroidism can mimic FM (see Step 3B: Replenish Nutrition for Organ, Gland or System Weakness, Thyroid).

Central Nervous System Disorders: "Raynaud's phenomenon" is highly correlated to FM. Raynaud's causes circulation problems of cold, possibly bluish, tingling, and burning arms and legs.

Gulf War Syndrome (GWS): Raynaud's and GWS have similar symptoms, and detoxing seems to help both immensely. Both have chemical exposure/vaccinations as suspected causes. In GWS, anti-squalene antibodies were found to be prevalent (squalene was a vaccination base).

Adrenals/pancreas: Many experience adrenal fatigue/hypoglycemia and need support.

Altered Neurotransmitters: Low serotonin levels are correlated to FM. Serotonin helps us sleep and dulls the perception of pain; muscle pain is much more exaggerated when serotonin is low. Epinephrine and norepinephrine, on the other hand, are associated with causing flare-ups, (Step 3A:Reset Adrenals) (Step 3B: Replenish Nutrition for Organ, Gland or System Weakness, Pancreas, Brain).

Other causes/triggers: (Step 3:) Lyme disease; CFS; anemia; heavy metal toxicity; (Step 1:) physical trauma or abuse; (Step 5:) emotional states; fatty acid deficiency; (Step 4:) food allergies; and yeast/bacterial/viral/parasitic infections can be contributing factors. Defective T-cell activation might also be suspect (see also Step 3C: Reduce Infective Organisms in the Body). **You get the idea: EACH OF THE SIX INTERFERENCES MUST BE EVALUATED AND TREATED WITH THE SIX STEPS TO WELLNESS, IN ORDER TO ACHIEVE OPTIMAL HEALTH!**

FURTHER STEP 3: NUTRIENT APPLICATIONS FOR FM

Regulate Cortisol Levels: Cortisol is a hormone that controls the activity level of the immune system. Too much cortisol leads to suppression of the immune system and too little allows the immune system to be overreactive. FM patients have low cortisol levels. Several nutrients, which help maintain healthy cortisol levels, include: phosphatidyl serine, phospatidylethanolamine, phosphatidylcholine and DMAE (see Step 3A: Adrenals, 3C: Immune System).

Detoxing (Step 6) and removing offending allergens (Step 4), toxins, immune complexes, metals and parasites can help in removing triggers. Immune complexes, that form with foreign antigens, are supposed to be cleared by the liver and other detox pathways. However a faulty detox system will allow these complexes to deposit in tissues, where they can trigger or aggravate existing FM. Additionally, St. Amand's theory states that FM patients have reduced ability to excrete phosphates (in healthy people, these phosphates are excreted by the kidneys), which are ubiquitous in the food we eat. The theory also states that the phosphates are accumulating in the energy-producing parts of the cell, namely the mitochondria. These phosphates then accumulate in other tissues and cause symptoms.

SAM-e (S-adenosylmethionine) has been shown, in some clinical trials, to reduce the number of trigger points and areas of pain, lessen pain and fatigue, and improve mood. Using the nutrients to facilitate the homocysteine pathway will foster the natural production of SAM-e, which is less expensive and more effective. It's also safer because, SAM turns into S-adenosyl-homocysteine in just one step and toxic homocysteine in one more. If you don't have all of the nutrients, to take the pathway to the end, it will not help to supplement with SAM! A synergistic formula, Homocysteine Redux™ is recommended, to address the whole pathway, namely one that contains the B vitamins, betaine, and methylating agents, such as folic acid, etc.

Calcium and magnesium are needed for muscle health, proper contraction-relaxations and healing of muscle fibers and muscle connective tissue. Magnesium was found to be efficacious in relieving muscle pain in an uncontrolled study, but not in a double-blind study (see Step 3: Joints). Vitamin E has had reputed benefits since early studies. One hundred to 300 IU daily resulted in positive, sometimes dramatic, benefits. FM patients exhibit a low Vitamin B-1 status and thus have reduced activity of thiamine-dependent enzymes. TPP, which is a thiamine-dependent enzyme, is critical for the energy-producing Kreb's cycle.

Symptoms of FM commonly include muscle fatigue and soreness with inflammation. For these symptoms, several nutrients and herbs may be helpful, such as: valerian, skullcap and passionflower, as they are all calming to the central nervous system. Feverfew is pain-relieving, and bromelain can help with inflammation. *Medicine and Science in Sports and Exercise* reports a study on bromelain, an enzyme that has "therapeutic effects in the treatment of inflammation and soft tissue injuries."

Anti-inflammatory herbs include ginger and turmeric. Ginger contains phenolic compounds that inhibit the enzymes responsible for generating important mediators of pain and inflammation in more than one pathway. Turmeric has demonstrated excellent anti-inflammatory and antioxidant properties, especially curcumin, which is the active component of turmeric that is responsible for the yellow pigment (see Step 3: Nutrition for Joints, Inflammation and Pain-Total Inflam™ and Total Joint Repair™).

Regular low-intensity exercise may improve symptoms of fibromyalgia. Patients report that they suffer less severe symptoms when on an exercise regimen. Acupuncture, adjustments, emotional release, detoxification, nutritional support, etc., can also help the symptoms of FM. The best regimen for addressing FM is to incorporate all 6 levels of treatment. In other words, in order to achieve optimal wellness, all Six Pieces of the Health Puzzle must be put together – in the right order – at the right time.

ENVIRONMENTAL ILLNESS

Toxins in our environment have accumulated and increased so rapidly, that it is increasingly difficult to identify a singular cause of disease. Dr. James Braly states, "Seriously allergic and sensitive people are essentially no different from everyone else — it's a difference in degree, not kind. Their suffering is a clear warning to the rest of us about the incredible invisible dangers of our surroundings."

Psychological disturbances can result from stored toxins within the central nervous system. Every body organ has a certain amount of fat in its composition; however, the brain and nervous tissue have an extremely high content, and that's the tissue where toxins get stored. Mercury has a particularly high affinity for brain and nervous tissue.

When not detoxified, chemicals, poisons and metals can interfere with the neurotransmitter pathways. A TV special focused on a prisoner who had been convicted of murder. He suffered all the signs of neurological dysfunction resulting from a chemical exposure to a heavy-duty insecticide containing poisons that inhibit a major neurotransmitter, acetylcholine. The murderer, who previously had been a model, law-abiding citizen, was exposed to this poison constantly on his job. After a long exposure one day, he exhibited signs of neurological toxicity, acted totally out of character and killed a complete stranger.

SICK BUILDING SYNDROME

Offending toxins range from smoke, dust/building material particles and microbials (molds, bacteria, fungi) to chemicals (paint, cleaning products, carpet gases, etc.). Harmful effects can include headaches, fatigue, dizziness, emphysema, rashes, respiratory distress, allergic reactions, chronic illness, etc. Ironically, learning impairment is one of the symptoms of "sick building syndrome," and yet schools can be one of the places harboring this risk.

For example, Malathion is a common household insecticide, which carries a caution on the label warning about liver damage. The most common danger is usually from chronic exposure of small amounts that build up in the liver. In 1999, however, a class-action suit was filed against the Malathion manufacturer, Cheminova, claiming personal and property damage to more than one million Florida residents, due to blanket spraying for mosquitoes.

ELECTROMAGNETIC FIELDS (EMFS) – STEP 2 REVISITED:

Invisible, active forces such as power lines, computers, kitchen appliances, tools, wiring, etc., can change biological tissue. Environmental sensitivity and individual tolerances are not measured when EMF studies are conducted, making it all the more difficult to reach significant test results. However, although this topic is highly debated, there is an immense amount of scientific literature that indicates EMFs can be a threat to our health.

Several studies have found associations between wire configuration codes and childhood cancer. In one study, a modified code was used to reanalyze data from a case-control study of childhood cancer in the Denver metropolitan area. This small change in coding generated risk estimates that were markedly elevated for the high-wire code and yielded odds ratios of 1:9 for total cancers, 2:9 for leukemias, and 2:5 for brain cancer that were not confounded by measured potential risk factors for childhood cancer.

SAUNA DETOXIFICATION

Sweat lodges have been used for centuries by, Native Americans, to help cleanse and purify the body and soul. Many European communities use them, routinely, as a way to relax and heal. Finnish people are known for popularizing sauna use. The Finns' ancient religious ceremonies used it for mental, spiritual and physical cleansing, a practice that dated from 5,000 and 3,000 BC from an area northwest of Tibet to their present location in Finland.

Improved technology now allows you to tolerate and benefit from this wonderful detox method at a much lower temperature. You get profuse sweating without burning eyes, and the skin does its work better to release toxins of all kinds. Modern technology produces heat from the new infrared saunas, such as the Thermal Life® unit (from High Tech Health, 1-800-794-5355). We use this unit at home and in the clinic. The infrared radiation is similar to the heat of the sun, but is not

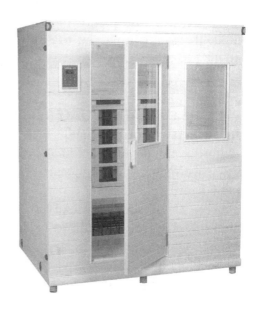

toxic like many artificially created electromagnetic fields.

In fact, Japanese research suggests that the heat of the infrared sauna also helps detoxify harmful radiation byproducts from artificial electromagnetic sources. It has been suggested that sweat is normally 2% toxins, but jumps to 15% toxins when induced by the High Tec far infrared sauna.

This new infrared technology produces radiation that is related to the wavelengths, produced by our body's own tissues that burn sugar and fat as fuel, to produce tissue repair and keep our bodies warm. This infrared technology can simply enhance a number of the body's natural healing activities. Dr. Chi has described this kind of positive infrared radiation as "tuned to the body's needs." The skin cells selectively absorb positive infrared energy in a phenomenon he calls, "resonant absorption."

Our own bodies radiate heat as infrared energy, through the skin and palms, at wavelengths of 3 to 50 microns. The Thermal Life® unit, in its infrared sauna, radiates one-third of its energy in the short infrared band (from 2 to 5.6 microns) for deep penetration, and the other two-thirds in the long band (5.6 to 25 microns.) This approximates a natural peak human output. Chinese research considers wavelengths between 2 to 25 microns optimally therapeutic.

The body can release toxins through the bowel, urine, breath and skin, especially through sweating. Of course, in this process, the body will lose plenty of water, harmful metals and essential minerals, so it's important to drink plenty of pure water to replace all the essential and protective minerals lost.

BREATHE PURE AIR, EXHALE TOXINS

An essay named, "Breathe," written for participants in Dr. Robert Fulford's craniosacral seminars, was first given to us years ago when we first learned the basic elements of his structural therapy. Dr. Fulford believed that the breath was fundamental to the health of all people. "Breathing enlivens and vitalizes the physical body with life energy," Dr. Fulford said, "and also balances the flow of life energy within the body."

The energizing source was believed to be the breath, as it was in esoteric writings, ionizing and giving life to all other systems of the body. With deep, relaxed breathing, we can accomplish many things: relaxation, release of tension, healthy sleep patterns, healthy mind, brain, nerves and body. He also emphasized that breathing must be done through the nose, not the mouth.

Any trauma, physical or emotional, stops the breath. Most people jam the breath as soon as they are stressed, exactly the reverse of what should happen. "The more our breath is freed up, the less the effect of the trauma," Fulford said. Most therapists have integrated deep voluntary breathing instructions into various techniques of releasing stress from the body and mind. They have made it an essential part of body work, craniosacral release, and other techniques of releasing tensions that may go back all the way to birthing, most of which were not all that gentle.

We work with structure to free the breathing process, on a number of levels, to release physical and emotional tensions from *Step 1: The Foundation of Health: Re-establish Structural Integrity,* throughout the process and in conjunction with *Step 5: Re-evaluate Emotional Patterns and Remove Limiting Belief Systems.*

Our elimination system needs to be fully operational for optimal health. As previously mentioned, 70% of our toxins are eliminated by breathing. If you can improve your breathing, you can improve your overall health and elimination of toxins.

INDOOR AIR QUALITY

Equally important to proper breathing is the quality of the air we take in. Dr. Toohey furnished us much more evidence of environmental toxins than we could print. Environmental Protection Agency studies of human exposure to air pollutants found that indoor levels of pollutants are 2-5 times, and occasionally more than 100 times, higher than outdoor levels. These levels of indoor air pollutants, may be of particular concern because most people spend about 90% of their time indoors.

Air pollution contributes to lung disease, including respiratory tract infections, asthma and lung cancer. Lung disease claims close to 335,000 lives in America every year and is the third-leading cause of death in the U.S. Poor indoor air quality can cause headaches, dry eyes, nasal congestion, nausea or fatigue.

Biological pollutants include molds, bacteria, viruses, pollen, dust mites and animal dander, and they promote poor indoor air quality. In office buildings, heating, cooling and ventilation systems are frequent sources of biological pollutants.

Environmental tobacco smoke, or "second-hand smoke," is a major indoor air pollutant. It contains about 4,000 chemicals, including 200 known poisons, such as formaldehyde and carbon monoxide, as well as 43 carcinogens. Second hand smoke is estimated to cause 3,000 lung cancer deaths and 35,000 to 50,000 heart disease deaths in non-smokers, as well as 150,000 to 300,000 cases of lower respiratory tract infections in children under 18 months of age, each year.

Formaldehyde is a common chemical that outgases from bonding agents in carpets, upholstery, particleboard and plywood paneling. Formaldehyde gas may cause coughing, eye, nose and throat irritation, skin rashes, headaches and dizziness.

Asbestos fibers are light and small enough to remain airborne. They can be inhaled into the lungs and cause scarring of the lung tissue, lung cancer, and a special cancer-mesothelioma, a cancer that affects the lining of the lung or abdominal cavity. Many asbestos products are found in roofing and flooring, wall and pipe insulation, spackling compounds, cement, coating materials, heating equipment and acoustic insulation. These products are a potential problem indoors, if the asbestos-containing material is disturbed and becomes airborne, or when it disintegrates with age.

Heating systems, stoves or fireplaces using gas, fuel or wood produce several combustion products, the most dangerous of which are carbon monoxide and nitrogen dioxide.

Household cleaning agents, personal care products, pesticides, paints, hobby products and solvents are sources of hundreds of potentially harmful chemicals. Many household and personal care products can cause dizziness, nausea, allergic reactions, eye-skin-respiratory tract irritation and cancer.

WATCHING OUR WATER

It has been estimated that up to three out of every five Americans will be infected by parasites at some point in their lives. Parasites, which are organisms that invade and feed off a host organism, can be responsible for a wide variety of illnesses, including Crohn's Disease, Ulcerative Colitis, Rheumatoid Arthritis, Chronic Fatigue Syndrome, Epstein Barr virus, Irritable Bowel Syndrome and digestive complaints.

Almost half the people suffering from irritable bowel syndrome have parasitic infestations, and most are cured when the parasites are treated. 80% percent of those suffering from chronic fatigue were relieved of their symptoms when they were treated for parasites.

We now have a new problem – second-hand drugs! Up to 90% of excreted drugs can remain biologically active. This is suspected of contributing to pathogens' ever-increasing resistance to antibiotic drugs. People have a habit of flushing their unused drugs down the toilet.

Our body is composed of 70% water. Water is important to nearly all bodily processes, from digestion, absorption and circulation, to transporting nutrients and excretion of bodily wastes and toxins. It's important to drink about eight 8-10 ounce glasses of water a day (adjusting as necessary based on temperature, exercise and climate).

WHAT'S IN MY H2O?

Pollutants from heavy metals, fertilizers, pesticides, herbicides, new road construction, asbestos and industrial chemicals may be in any tap-water source. Other pollutants are deliberately added to public water supplies. Chlorine, aluminum sulfate, phosphates, soda ash, carbon and/or lime are added to kill bacteria, eliminate cloudiness and adjust pH. Though intended to be protectants, parasites aren't always killed by these additions.

When chlorine levels are high, chlorine byproducts produce known cancer-causing agents. Pesticide residues in tap water are known carcinogens as well, being composed of artificial compounds that mimic estrogen. In agricultural areas and in locations that were in former agricultural areas, this has been found to be a major problem. Remnants of pesticides persist for decades. Cryptosporidium, a parasite that can be fatal to immune-compromised individuals, is also commonly found in areas where water is polluted by agricultural runoff.

In 1961, *The Congressional Record* exposed artificial fluoride, which is added to our water supplies, as a lethal poison. In its natural form as calcium fluoride, fluoride is non-toxic. But in the forms recycled from industry and deliberately added to our public water supplies, fluoride has been linked with mottled teeth, brittle bones in old age, Down's Syndrome and cancer. Fluoride is commonly used as a rat poison and insecticide.

Unfortunately, water supplies are still artificially fluoridated in many localities, and foods and drinks in fluoridated areas contain fluoride. When these sources are added together with the fluoride found in conventional toothpastes, it adds up to a potential danger to our health.

IS BOTTLED WATER BETTER?

Since some states have no rules governing truth in labeling, it's difficult, if not impossible, to tell from the bottle's label.

If you use water from a water cooler at work or home, be sure to clean and disinfect the cooler by running a 50/50 solution of hydrogen peroxide and baking soda through the spigots and reservoir once a month.

HOW TO IMPROVE TAP WATER

Micro-filtration filters, with ion-exchange systems, help remove heavy metals. Reverse-osmosis systems are generally considered good, and systems that combine various methods of filtration are considered best.

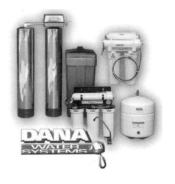

We recommend the water filtration system that we use in our homes: The Dana Water System. (www.danawater.com, 480-396-4778). The company custom makes each system to purify your specific water. You send in a sample of your water and the unit is made especially for your needs. They will keep your water at a pH of 7, which is optimal. Most water systems are much more acid and it is hard for your body to stay alkaline enough.

SUMMARY

- Toxins are a serious environmental health hazard. Toxic metals are widely used in industry, food processing and agriculture and are in our air, food and water.
- A whole-food, high-fiber diet helps toxins pass without entering your system.
- Breathing properly, vegetable-brush skin rubs and 20-minute baths with Epsom salt and baking soda (or Epsom salt and ginger) facilitates toxin elimination from the body.
- It is important to remove parasites that weaken the entire system.
- Detoxification, mineral balance, plenty of fluids and exercise are all important for good health.
- Homeopathic remedies help trigger the release of heavy-metal poisoning from your body through the breath, skin, urine or feces.
- Cold laser treatment and frequency modulation may increase blood and lymph circulation, helping remove toxins from the tissues.

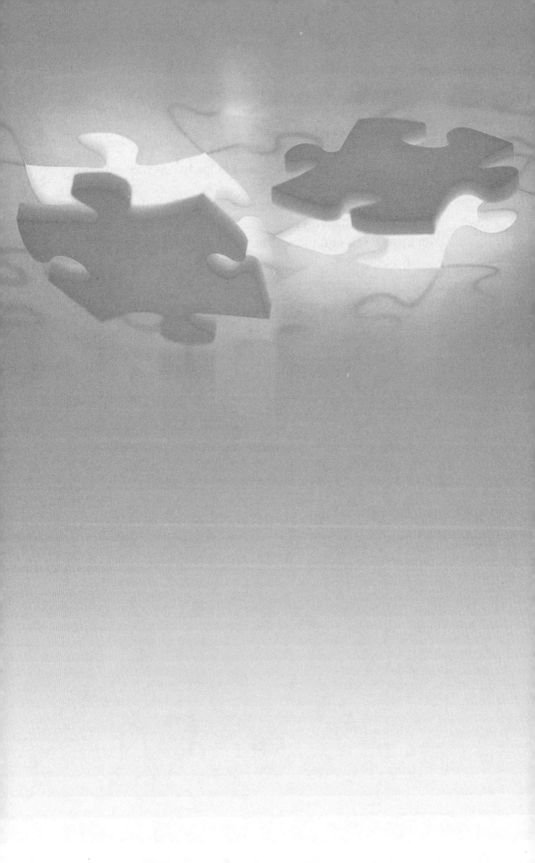

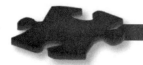

A FINAL THOUGHT

To say this book and its contents are controversial is an understatement. What we do in our offices is not possible by standard thought and protocol. If we had listened to what was accepted as usual and customary, there would be thousands of patients around the world who wouldn't be helped every single day.

According to science and measurement, a hummingbird and a bumblebee can't fly; it is aerodynamically impossible. So, does that mean the hummingbird and bumblebee have to stop flying until science can figure out how they do it? We all see the answer to that question every day. They do fly, and they will fly, and do it very well.

Like the hummingbird and the bumblebee, we embrace our own reality. We are going to continue to do the impossible until science can catch up with us to explain it. Will we be heralded as geniuses at that time? We think not. But, that's not what's important to us. **What's important to us is helping people help themselves**. "We, the Few" who dare to challenge dogma and seek truth, wherever we can find it, do it to give people hope and help where it didn't exist within the box of conventional science and medicine.

We don't go outside the box just to be different. We go outside to make a difference. If people would have gained the level of wellness they sought, staying inside the box, we would have been happy to stay there as well. "Illness" is not caused by drug deficiencies. Colds are not caught - they're earned. We cannot name and blame illness and then cover its symptoms with drugs and surgery, pretending we were just victims.

THE FIRST DAY and EVERY DAY CAN MAKE A DIFFERENCE!

When all 6 avenues of interference are explored, evaluated and removed, and the Pieces of the Health Puzzle are put together, the body will most often return to wellness. The body is a miracle, and we truly do See Miracles Daily in our office.

By removing the 6 Interferences to Health with the 6 Steps to Wellness, we are able to allow the innate intelligence that created the body – heal the body. The 6 Steps to Wellness is not just an answer...it has been the **ONLY ANSWER** for many, and may be the answer for you!

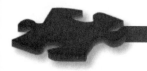

REFERENCES BY CHAPTER

Step 1: The Foundation of Health: Re-Establish Structural Integrity

"Assistance in liposuction appears effective, low-level lasers warrant study," Dermatology Times Jan 2003; 24(1).

"Speed healing: low-level laser heals wounds quicker," Dermatology Times Dec 2002; 23(12).

Altman, N., Everybody's Guide to Chiropractic Health Care, Los Angeles: Jeremy P. Tarcher, Inc, 1990.

Al-Watban, F.A.H. and Andres, B.L., "Laser photons and pharmacological treatments in wound healing," Laser Therapy Special Millennium Edition 2000; 12:3-11.

Al-Watban F.A.H. and Delgado, "Erchonia laser (635nm) on healing of scalpel wound on rats," Laser Medicine Section, Biological and Medical Research Dept, King Faisal Specialist Hospital and Research Centre, Riyadh, Saudi Arabia, unpublished article submitted to Lasers and Surgery in Medicine.

Amy, R. et al, "Does the frequency of Pulse laser play any role in pain reduction in humans," An abstract of the Erchonia LASER clinical trial, July Sept 2000: 1-5.

Amy, R., The Low Level Laser Protocol Book, Therapeutic Laser Applications for Injury Management and Peripheral-Central Nervous System Regulation, Top Ten Laser Protocols, A to Z Protocols, n.d.: 1-37.

Asagai, Y. et al, "Thermographic study of low level laser therapy for acute-phase injury," Laser Therapy Special Millennium Edition 2000; 12:31-33.

Berkson, D.L., "Osteoarthritis, Chiropractic, and Nutrition: Osteoarthritis considered as a natural part of a three stage subluxation complex: its reversibility: its relevance and treatability by chiropractic and nutritional correlates," Medical Hypotheses 1991; (36):356-67.

Bremiller, W.S., "Laser use for pain and healing in athletic medicine," Physical Therapy Forum 3 July 1985; IV(26):1,3.

Castel, J.C., "Pain management and acupuncture, TENS, and photostimulation," Lake Bluff, Pain Control Services, Inc 1982.

Enwemeka, C.S. and Reddy, G.K., "The biological effects of laser therapy and other physical modalities on connective tissue repair processes," Laser Therapy Special Millennium Edition 2000; 12:22-30.

Fryman, V.M., "A study of the rhythmic motions of the living cranium," J. of the Am Osteopath Assoc May 1971(70): 928-45.

Fulford, R.C. and Stone, G., Dr. Fulford's Touch of Life: The Healing Power of the Natural Life Force, NY: Pocket Books, 1996.

Fulford, R.C., "Breath," Seminar Publication, 1991.

Glazewski, J., "The special application of low intensity lasers to rheumatology—results of four-year observations of 224 patients," European Biomedical Optics Week BIOS Europe '96. Abstract Book 1996, 96. Vienna.

Glazewski, J.B., "Low-energy laser therapy as quantum medicine," Laser Therapy Special Millennium Edition 2000; 12: 39-42.

Gur A. et al, "Effects of low power laser and low dose amitriptyline therapy on clinical symptoms and quality of life in fibromyalgia: a single-blind, placebo-controlled trial," Rheumatol Int Sep 2002;22(5):188-93.

Ho, M.W., The Rainbow and the Worm, The Physics of Organisms, 2nd Edition, River Edge, NJ: World Scientific Publishing, 1998.

Horwitz, L.R. et al, "Augmentation of wound healing using monochromatic infrared energy," Advances in Wound Care Jan Feb 1999; 12(1):35-40.

Jarvis, K.B. et al, "Cost per case comparison of back injury claims: Chiropractic versus medical management for conditions with identical analysis codes," J. of Occupational Med Aug 1991; 33(8): 847-52.

Kleinkort, J. and Foley, R., "Laser: a preliminary report on its use in physical therapy," Clinical Management in Physical Therapy Winter 1982; 2(4): 30-2.

Kovinski, I.T., "The treatment of burns by laser," Zdravoohr

Kaz 1973; 3:46.

Lubart, R. et al, "Photobiological stimulation as a function of different wavelengths," Laser Therapy Special Millennium Edition 2000; 12:38-41.

Mester et al, "Stimulation of wound healing by laser rays," Acta Chirugica Academiae Scientarum Hungaricae 1972; 13(3): 315-27.

Moreno, C., "Ultra structure of mitochondrions after laser microirradiation," Journal de Microscopic 1973; 16(3): 269-279.

Navratil, L. and Dylevsky, I., "Mechanisms of the analgesic effect of therapeutic lasers in vivo," Laser Therapy 1997; 9:33-39.

Neira, R. et al, "Fat liquefaction: effect of low-level laser energy on adipose tissue," Plastic and Reconstructive Surgery Sept 2002; 110(3): 912-22.

Neira, R. et al, "Low-level laser-assisted lipoplasty appearance of fat demonstrated by MRI on abdominal tissue," Am J of Cosmetic Surgery 2001; 18(3):133-140.

Oschman, Energy Medicine in Therapeutics and Human Performance, NY: Butterworth Heinemann, 2003.

Pascu, M.L., "Laser physics elements to consider for low level laser therapy," Laser Therapy Special Millennium Edition 2001; 13:114-125.

Reich, W., Selected Writings. NY: Farrar, Straus and Giroux, 1971.

Reiman, P., "Laser-assisted liposuction aids wound healing," Cosmetic Surgery Times June 2002; 5(5).

Rochkind, S. and Quaknine, G.E., "New trend in neuroscience: low-power laser effect on peripheral and central nervous system (basic science, preclinical and clinical studies)," Neurological Research March 1992; 14:2-11.

Rochkind, S. et al, "Effects of laser irradiation on the spinal cord for the regeneration of crushed peripheral nerve in rats," Lasers in Surgery and Medicine 2001; 28:216-19.

Rochkind, S. et al, "New method of treatment of severely injured sciatic nerve and spinal cord: an experimental study," Acta Neurochir Suppl (Wein) 1988; 43: 91-3.

Rochkind, S. et al, "Response of He-Ne laser: experimental studies," Laser Surg Med 1987; 7: 441-43.

Rochkind, S. et al, "Stable severe spinal cord and cauda

equine injury or damage: results of laser treatment," Laser Bologna '92, 3rd World Congress, International Society for Low Power Laser Applications in Medicine, Sept 9-12 1992: 71-75.

The Burton Goldberg Group, Alternative Medicine, The Definitive Guide, Fife, Washington: Future Medicine Publishing, Inc., 1995; "Chiropractic," 134-142.

Upledger, J.E., Your Inner Physician and You, craniosacral therapy and SomatoEmotional Release. Berkeley, CA: North Atlantic, 1992.

Weil, A., Natural Health, Natural Medicine: A Comprehensive Guide to Wellness and Self-Care. Boston, MA: Houghton Mifflin, 1990.

Weil, A., Spontaneous Healing. NY: Random House, 1995.

Wong, E. et al, "Successful management of female office workers with "repetitive stress injury" or "carpal tunnel

Worcester, S., "Low-level laser could 'revolutionize' liposuction," Skin and Allergy News May 2002; 33(5).

Step 2: Rebalance Electromagnetics

Becker, R.O., The Promise of Electromedicine, The Perils of Electropollution, Los Angeles, Jeremy P Tarcher, 1990; Chapter 3, The New Scientific Revolution; Chapter 7, The Natural Electromagnetic Field; Chapter 8, Man-Made Electromagnetic fields; Chapter 9, Elf and the Mind/Brain Problem; Chapter 11, The New Plagues; Chapter 12, The Risk and Benefits, What You Can Do.

"Biological effects of power line fields, Final report of the New York State Dept of Health, Scientific Advisory Board, July 1, 1987.

Brown, H.D. et al, "A review of scientific literature on electropollution," Cancer Biochem Society and Biophysics 1988; (9): 295.

Step 3 Rebuild With Nutrition
3A): Rest Adrenals & the General Adaptive Syndrome (GAS)

Balch, J.F. and Balch, P.A., Prescription for Nutritional Healing, 2nd Edition, New York: Avery, 1997.

Campbell, T.A., "Study on diet, nutrition and disease in the Peoples Republic of China, Part II," Revision of Nutritional Science, Cornell University, Ithaca, New York, 1985.

Carper, J., The Food Pharmacy, New York: Bantam Books, 1988.

Chaitow, L., Amino Acids in Therapy, Rochester, Vermont: Healing Arts Press, 1988.

International College of Applied Kinesiology, Collected Papers, Winter Meeting, 1977: 21.

Lininger, S., Wright, J., Austin, S., Brown, D., Gaby. A., The Natural Pharmacy, Rocklin, CA: Prima Health, 1998.

Mindell, E., Earl Mindell's Vitamin Bible, New York: Warner Books, 1991.

National Center for Health Statistics, Health United States, 1989 DHHS publication, 90-1232. U.S. Government printing office, Washington, D.C., 1990: 108.

Ornish, D., Stress, Diet and Your Heart, New York: Holt, Rinehart, and Winston Publishers, 1982.

Rector-Page, L., How to be Your Own Herbal Pharmacist, An Herbal Formula Reference, Sierra Foothills, CA: Crystal Star, 1991.

Schutte, K.H., and Myers JA, Metabolic Aspects of Health, Kentfield, CA: Discovery Press, 1979.

Selye, H., Stress Without Distress, New York, NY: The New American Library, Inc, 1975.

Sorenson, M, Mega Health, Ivins, UT: NIF: 370-392.
Step 3: Reset Adrenals to Combat G.A.S.

The Burton Goldberg Group, Alternative Medicine, The Definitive Guide, Fife, Washington: Future Medicine Publishing, Inc., 1995

Warning: Hostility can be dangerous to your health. University of Texas, Lifetime Health Letter, Oct. 1989.

Step 3B): Replenish Nutrition For Organ, Gland Or System Weakness

"Silicon and Bone Formation," *Nutr Rev* 1980; 38: 194-195.

"Two Studies Indicate Vitamin D Metabolite Curbs Osteoporosis," *Family Pract News* March 1984; 15: 2. 1985;703:225-33.

Anonymous, "Biotin and glucokinase in the diabetic rat nutrition," *Rev* 1970; 28:242-244

Arruzazabala, M.L. et al, "Effect of policosanol on cerebral ischemia in Mongolian gerbils: Role of prostacyclin and thromboxane," *Az Prostaglandins Leuko Essent Fatty Acids* 1993; (49):695-697.

Asayama, K., Koony, N.W., and Burr, I.M., "Effect of Vitamin E. Deficiency and selenium deficiency on insulin secretory reserve and free radical scavenging systems in islets: Decrease of islet manganosuperoxide dismutase," *J Lab Clin Med* 1986; 107:459-464.

Balch and Balch 1990: 241.

Balch, J.F. and Balch, P.A., *Prescription for Nutritional Healing,* 2nd and 3rd Editions, New York: Avery, 1997, 2000.

Bazzato, G., "Myasthenia-like Syndrome After DL- but not L-Carnitine," *Lancet* 1981;1: 1209.

Berkow, R., *The Merck Manual,* 16th Ed., Rathway, NJ: Merck Research Laboratories, 1992.

Beyer, R.B., "Inhibition by Coenzyme Q of Ethanol and Carbon Tetrachloride-Stimulated Lipid Peroxidation in Vivo and Catalyzed by Mitochondrial Systems," *Free Radical Biology and Medicine* 1985; 5: 297-303.

Biggs, B.L., Melton LJ III, "Involutional Osteoporosis," *N Engl J Med* 1986; 314: 1676-1686.

Bliznakov, E., Hunt, G., *The Miracle Nutrient Coenzyme Q10,* New York: Bantam, 1987.

Bone Thinning in Postmenopausal Women With Primary Biliary Cirrhosis," *Am J Clin Nutr* 1982; 36: 426-430.

Bordia, A.K., "The Effect of Vitamin C on Blood Lipids, Fibrinolytic Activity and Platelet Adhesiveness in Patients with Coronary Artery Disease," *Atherosclerosis* 1980; 35: 181-187.

Burton Goldberg Group, *Alternative Medicine, The Definitive Guide,* Fife, Washington: Future Medicine Publishing, 1995.

Cameron, E. and Pauling, L., "Supplemental Ascorbate in the Supportive Treatment of Cancer. Prolongation of Survival Times in Terminal Human Cancer," *Proc National Academy of Science* 1982; 73: 3685.

Carli, P. et al, *Presse Med* 1995; 24:606-610.

Carper, J., *The Food Pharmacy, Dramatic New Evidence that Food is Your Best Medicine,* New York: Bantam, 1989.

Cats, A. et al, "Effect of frequent consumption of a Lactobacillus casei-containing milk drink in Helicobacter pylori-colonized subjects," *Aliment Pharmacol Ther* Feb 2003;17(3):429-35.

Cavallo, et al, *The Lancet* 1996; 348:926-928.

Chaitow L, *Amino Acids in Therapy,* Rochester, Vermont: Healing Arts Press, 1988.

Christiane, N., *Women's Bodies, Women's Wisdom [sic}.*
Cien Biol 1991; (22): 62-63.

Coggeshall, J.C., Heggars, J.P., Robson, M.C., Baker. H., "Biotin status and plasma glucose in diabetics," *Ann NY Acad Sci* 1985; 447:389-393.

Cordain, L., Toohey, L., Smith, M.J., Hickey MS, "Modulation of Immune Function by Dietary Lectins/Proteins in Rheumatoid Arthritis," *British Journal of Nutrition* April 2000; 83:207-217.

Cordain, L., Toohey, L., Smith, M.J., Hickey, M.S., "Modulation of Immune Function by Dietary Lectins/Proteins in Rheumatoid Arthritis," *British Journal of Nutrition* April 2000; 83:207-217.

Cordova, C., "Influence of Ascorbic Acid on Planet Aggregation in Vitro and In Vivo," *Atherosclerosis* 1982; 41: 15-19.

Crespo, N. et al, "Effect of policosanol on patients with non-insulin-dependent diabetes mellitus and hypercholesterolemia: A pilot study," *Curr Ther Res* 1997; (58): 44-51.

Cruz Bustillo, D. et al, "Efecto hipocolesterol mico del Ateromixol (PPG) en el cerdo en ceba," *Rev CENIC*
Cutler, E.W., *Winning the War Against Asthma and Allergies, A Drug-Free Cure for Asthma and Allergy Suffers,* Albany, New York: Delmar Publishers, 1998.

D'Adamo, P. and Whitney, C., *Eat Right for Your Type*, New York: G.P. Putnam's Sons, 1996: 53, 57, 72.

Davis, B., *Wellness Advocate* Feb 1995; 5(1):1-4).

Dipalma, J.R., "Carnitine Deficiency," *American Family Physician* 1988; 38:243-251.

Dolkers, K., Vadhanavikit, S., and Mortensen, S.A., "Biochemical Rationale and Myocardial Tissue Data on the Effective Therapy of Cardiomyopathy with coenzyme Q10," *Proc National Academy of Science* 1985; 62: 901-904.

Draper, C.R. et al, *J Nutr* 1997; 127:1795-99.

Durance, R.A. et al, "Treatment of Osteoporotic Patients. A Trail of Calcium Supplements and Ashed Bone," *Clin. Trials* 1973; 3: 67-73.

Eck, P.C., Wilson, L., *Toxic Metal in Human Health and Disease,* Phoenix, AZ: The Eck Institute of Applied Bioenergetics, Ltd., 1989.

Eckhert, C.D., Breskin, M.W., Wise, W.W., Knopp, R.H., "Association between low serum selenium and diminished visual function in diabetic women," *Fed Proc* 1985:44:1970.

Enan, G. et al, "Inhibition of Listeria monocytogenes LMG10470 by plantaricin UG1 in vitro and in beef meat," *Nahrung* Dec 2002;46(6):411-4.

Epstein, O. et al, "Vitamin D, Hydroxyapatite, and Calcium Gluconate in Treatment of Corticol.

Ferrari, R., Cacchini, F., and Visioli, O., "The Metabolic Effects of L-Carnitine in Angina Pectoris," *International Journal of Cardiology* 1984; 5: 213.

Flannery, G.R. et al, "Antimitochondrial antibodies in primary biliary cirrhosis recognize both specific peptides and shared epitopes of the M2 family of antigens," *Hepatology* 1989 Sep;10(3):370-4.

Flynn, S. et al, "Characterization of the genetic locus responsible for the production of ABP-118, a novel bacteriocin produced by the probiotic bacterium Lactobacillus salivarius subsp. salivarius UCC118," *Microbiology* Apr 2002;148 (Pt 4):973-84.

Follis, R.H. Jr. et al, "Studies on copper metabolism XVIII. Skeletal changes associated with copper deficiency in swine," *John Hopkins Hosp Bull* 1955; 97: 405-409.

Fraga, V. et al, "Effect of policosanol on in vivo and in vitro rat liver microsomal lipid peroxidation," *Arch Medical Res* 1997; (28): 355-360.

Franke et al, 1994.

Frithiof, L. et al, "The relationship between marginal bone loss and serum zinc levels," *Acta Med Scand* 1980; 207: 67-70.

Gaby, A,R, and Wright, J.V., *The Patient's Book of Natural Healing,* Rocklin, CA: Prima Health Book, 1999.

Gallagher, J.C., Riggs, B.L., DeLuca, H.F., "Effect of treatment with synthetic 1:25-dihydroxy Vitamin D in postmenopausal osteoporosis," *Clin Res* 1979; 27: 366A.

Gallop, P.M., Lian, J.B., Hauschka, P.V., "Carboxylated calcium-binding proteins and Vitamin K," *N Eng J Med* 1980; 302: 1460-1466.

Gard, Z.R. et al.,*Explore for the Professional,* 1995;6 (4):39-45.

Gastroenterology 1974; 67:531-50.

Glick, L., *Lancet* 1982; ii: 817

Glinsmann, W.H., Mertz, W., "Effect of trivalant chromium on glucose metabolism," 1966; 15:502-510.

Hall, J.C. et al, *Br J Surg* Mar 1996; 83(3): 305-312.

Hargrove, J. et al., "Menopausal Hormone Replacement Therapy with Continuous Daily Oral Micronized Estradiol and Progesterone," *Obstetrics and Gynecology* 1989; 73:606 as cited in Ojeda L, *Menopause without Medicine* Alameda CA: Hunter House Publ, 1989: 107.

Head, K.A., "Inositol hexaniacinate: a safer alternative to niacin," *Alt Med Rev* 1996; (1): 176-84.

Heany, R.P., "Thinking Straight About Calcium," *N Eng J Med* 1993; 328(7): 503-505.

Heres, L. et al, "Fermented liquid feed reduces susceptibility of broilers for Salmonella enteritidis," *Poult Sci* Apr 2003;82(4):603-11.

Hobbs, C., *Medicinal Mushrooms,* Santa Cruz, CA: Botanica Press, 1996.

Hoorfar, J. et al., Diabetes Research. 1992;20:33-41, p. 38.

Hori, T. et al, "Effect of an oral administration of Lactobacillus casei strain Shirota on the natural killer activity of blood mononuclear cells in aged mice," *Biosci Biotechnol*

Biochem Feb 2003;67(2):420-2. human fibroblasts," *Bio Res* 1994; (27):199-203.

Hunt, C.D., Nielsen, F.H., "Interaction Between Boron and Cholecalciferol in the Chick," Hawthorne, J.M., Howell, J.M., and White, C.L., eds. *Trace Element Metabolism in Man and Animals,* Berlin, Springer-Verlag, 1982: 597-600.

Husby, S. et al, *Scand J Immunol* 1985; 22:83-92.

Ishiuama, T., Morita, Y., and Toyama, S., "A Clinical Study of the Effect of Coenzyme Q on Congestive Heart Failure*,"* *Japanese Heart Journal* 1978; 17:32.

J Nutr 1997; 127:1795-99

Jacob, S. et al, "Enhancement of glucose disposal in patients with type 2 diabetes by alpha-lipoic acid," *Arzneimittelforschung* 1995 Aug; 45(8):872 4.

JAMA July 17, 2002

Jayanthi, S.A.U., Jayanthi, G.A.U., Varalakshmi, P.T.I., "Effect of DL alpha-lipoic acid on some carbohydrate metabolizing enzymes in stone forming rats," *Biochem Int* 1991 Sep; 25(1):123-36.

Johnston, C. et al, "Calcium Supplementation and Increase in Bone Density in Children," *N Eng J Med* 1992; 327: 82-87.

Juarez, Tomas, MS et al, "Influence of pH, temperature and culture media on the growth and bacteriocin production by vaginal Lactobacillus salivarius CRL 1328," *J Appl Microbiol* 2002;93(4):714-24.

Kagan, V.E. et al, "Recycling of Vitamin E in human low density lipoproteins," *J Lipid Res* 1992 Mar; 33(3):385-97.

Kassir, Z.A., *Irish Med J* 1985; 78:153-56.

Kimber, D., Gary. C., and Stackpole, C.E., *Anatomy and Physiology.* New York: McMillan, 1996: 440-469.

Lark, S., *Fibroid tumors and Endometriosis*, Berkeley, CA: Celestial Arts, 1995: 125.

Lehninger, A., *Principles of Organic Chemistry*, New York: Worth, 1982; chaps. 14-17.

Leibovitz, B. and Siegel, B.V., "Ascorbic Acid, Neutrophil Function and the Immune Response," *International Journal of Vitamin and Nutrition* 1978; 48: 159.

Leibovitz, B., *Carnitine, the Vitamin BT Phenomenon,* New York: Dell, 1984.

Ley, B.M., *The Potato Antioxidant, Alpha Lipoic Acid,* New York: BL Publications, 1998.

Lininger S., editor in chief, Wright J, Austin S, Brown D, Gaby A, *The Natural Pharmacy,* Rocklin, CA: Prima Publishing, 1998.

Magnusson, J. et al, "Broad and complex antifungal activity among environmental isolates of lactic acid bacteria," *FEMS Microbiol Lett* Feb 2003 14;219(1):129-3.

Maitra, I. et al, "Alpha-lipoic acid prevents buthionine sulfoximine-induced cataract formation in newborn rats," *Free Radic Biol Med* 1995 Apr; 18(4):823-9.

Marcia Stefanick, chair of the Women's Health Initiative's Steering committee; *Newsweek* July 22, 2002:38-41.

McCaslin, F.E. Jr., Janes, J.M., "The Effect of Strontium Lactate in the Treatment of Osteoporosis," *Proc Staff Meetings Mayo Clin* 1959; 34: 329-334.

Medalle, R., Waterhouse, C., Hahn, T.J., "Vitamin D Resistance in Magnesium Deficiency," *Am J Clin Nutr* 1976; 29: 854-858.

Menindez, R., et al, "Policosanol inhibits cholesterol biosynthesis and enhances LDL processing in cultured

Mills, T..J, et al, "The Use of a Whole Bone Extract in the Treatment of Fractures," *Manitoba Medical Review* 1995; 45: 92-96.

Mindell, E., *Earl Mindell's Vitamin Bible,* New York: Warner Books, 1991.

Morgan, K.J., Stampley, G.L., Zabik, M.E., Fischer, D.R., "Magnesium and calcium dietary intakes of the U.S. population," *J Am Coll Nut* 1985; 4:195-206

Morgan, M.Y., "Hepatoprotective agents in alcoholic liver disease," *Acla Med Scand* Suppl

Mowrey, D.B., *The Scientific Validation of Herbal Medicine,* Cormorant Books, 1986 as cited by Lieberman S, *Journal of Women's Health* 1998; 7(5):525-529.

Murray, M., "Lipid lowering drugs vs. inositol hexaniacinate," *Am J Natural Med* 1995; (2): 9-12.

Murray, M., *Menopause*, Rocklin, CA: 1994.

Murray, M.T., *Natural Alternatives to Over-the-Counter*

and Prescription Drugs, NY: William Morrow and Company, Inc, 1994.

Nagamatsu, M. et al, "Lipoic acid improves nerve blood flow, reduces oxidative stress, and improves distal nerve conduction in experimental diabetic neuropathy," *Diabetes Care* 1995 Aug; 18(8):1160-7.

NE J Medicine, Sept 28 1995; 333(13): 839-844. ....

Newsweek, "Gut Reactions," November 17, 1997: 95-99.

Nielsen, E.M. et al, "Microcystalline Hydroxyapatite Compound in Corticosteroid Treated Rheumatoid Patients: A Controlled Study," *Brit Med J* 1978; 2: 1124.

Noa, M., Herrera, M., Magrancr, J., and Mas, R., "Effect of policosanol on isoprenaline-induced myocardial necrosis in rats," *J Pharm Pharmacol* 1994; (46):282-285.

Notoya, K. et al, *Calcif Tissue Int* 1992;51 (1): S3-S6.

Null, G., *The Woman's Encyclopedia of Natural Healing*, NY, NY: Seven Stories Press, 1996

O'Neill, C.A. et al, "Aldehyde-induced protein modifications in human plasma: protection by glutathione and dihydrolipoic acid," *J Lab Clin Med* 1994 Sep; 124 (3): 359 70.

Ozawa, H. et al, *Bone and Mineral* 1992; 19 (1): S21-S26

Packer, L. et al, "Alpha-Lipoic acid as a biological antioxidant," *Free Radic Biol Med* 1995 Aug; 19(2):227-50.

Packer, L., "Antioxidant properties of lipoic acid and its therapeutic effects in prevention of diabetes complications and cataracts," *Ann NY Acad Sci* 1994 Nov 17; 738:257-64.

Pauling, L., "Evolution and the Need for Ascorbic Acid," *Proc National Academy of Science* 1970; 67: 1643-1648.

Payne, S. et al, "In vitro studies on colonization resistance of the human gut microbiota to Candida albicans and the effects of tetracycline and Lactobacillus plantarum LPK," *Curr Issues Intest Microbiol* Mar 2003;4(1):1-8.

Pearson, D. and Shaw, S., *Life Extension*, New York: Warner Books, 1982.

Pennington, J.A.T. et al, *J Am Diet Assoc*, 86: 1986.

Pfeiffer, C.C., *Zinc and Other Micronutrients*, New Canaan, CN: Keats Publishing Co., 1978.

Pines, A. et al, "Clinical Trial of MCHC in the Prevention of

Osteoporosis Due to Corticosteroid Therapy," _Curr Med Res_ 1984; 8(10): 734-742.

Ransberger, K., "Enzyme Treatment of Immune Complex Disease," _Arthritis and Rheumatism_ 1986; 8: 16-19.

Rector-Page, L., _How to be Your Own Herbal Pharmacist, An Herbal Formula Reference,_ Sierra Foothills, CA: Crystal Star, 1991.

Riggs, B.L. et al, "Rates of Bone Loss in the Appendicular and Axial Skeletons of Women," _J Clin Invest_ 1986; 7: 1487-1491.

Rodgers, S. et al, "Inhibition of nonproteolytic Clostridium botulinum with lactic acid bacteria and their bacteriocins at refrigeration temperatures," _J Food Prot_ Apr 2003;66(4):674-8.

Sarji, K.E., Kleinfelder, J., Brewington, P., Gonzales, J., Hempling, H., "Decreased platelet Vitamin C in diabetes mellitus: Possible role in hyperaggregation," _Thromb Res_ 1979; 15:639-650.

Schroeder, H.A., Nason, A.P., Tipton, I.H., "Chromium Deficiency as a factor in arteriosclerosis," _J Chronic Dis_ 1970; 23:123-142.

Schwarzbein, D. and Deville, N., _The Schwarzbein Principle, The Truth About Losing Weight, Being Healthy and Feeling Younger,_ Deerfield Beach, FL: Health Communications, Inc, 1999.

Schwarzbein, D. with Brown, M., _The Schwarzbein Principle II, The Transition, A Regeneration Process to Prevent and Reverse Accelerated Aging,_ Deerfield Beach, FL: Health Communications, Inc, 2002.

Scott, F.W. et al, _Diabetes Res_, 1988; 7:153-157.

Sindhu, S.C. and Khetarpaul, N., "Effect of probiotic fermentation on antinutrients and in vitro protein and starch digestibilities of indigenously developed RWGT food mixture," _Nutr Health_ 2002;16(3):173-81.

Smith, C.J., "Non-hormonal control of vaso-motor flushing in menopausal patients," _Chicago Medicine_ March 7, 1964.

Smith, R.T., Smith, J.C., Fields, M., Reiser, S., "Mechanical Properties of Bone from Copper Deficient Rats Fed Starch or Fructose," Fed Proc 1985; 44: 541.

Stellon, A. et al, "Microcystalline Hydroxyapatite Compound in Prevention of Bone Loss In Corticosteroid-Treated Patients with Chronic Active Hepatitis," _Postgrad Med J_ 1985; 61: 791-796.

Stepan, J.J. et al, "Prospective Trial of Ossein-Hydroxyapatite Compound in Surgically Induced Postmenopausal Women," *Bone* 1989; 10: 179-185.

Stusser, R. et al, "Long-term therapy with policosanol improves treadmill exercise-ECG testing performance of coronary heart disease patients," *Int J Clin Pharmacol Ther* 1998; 36(9):469-73.

The Merck Manual, 16th Edition, R Berkow, editor in chief, et al., Rathway, NJ: Merck Research Laboratories, 1992.

Tierra, M., *The Way of Herbs, With the Latest Developments in Herbal Science,* New York: Pocket Books, 1990.

Toepfer, E.W., Mertz, W., Polansky, M.M., Roginski, E.E., "Preparation of chromium containing material of glucose tolerance factor activity from brewer's yeast extracts and by synthesis," *J Agric Food Chem* 1977; 25:162-166.

Toohey, L., "The Nutritional Connection to "Leaky Gut," *Am Chiropractor* Apr 2002.

Turchet, P. et al, "Effect of fermented milk containing the probiotic Lactobacillus casei DN-114 001 on winter infections in free-living elderly subjects: a randomized, controlled pilot study," *J Nutr Health Aging* 2003;7(2):75-7.

Valdes, S. et al, "Effect of policosanol on platelet aggregation in healthy volunteers," *Intern J Clin Pharmacol Res* 1996; (16): 67-72.

Werbach, M.R., M.D. *Nutritional Influences on Illness.* Tarzana, CA: Third Line Press, 1996.

Westin, J. and Richter, E., *Ann NY Acad Sci* 1990; 609:269-279.

Whitaker, J., *Dr. Whitaker's Guide to Natural Healing,* Prima Publishing, Rockline, CA, 1994: 310-316.

Wilson, T., Katz, J.M., Gray, D.H., "Inhibition of Active Bone Resorption by Copper," *Calcif Tissue Int* 1981; 33:35-39.

Windsor, A.C.M. et al, "The Effect of Whole Bone Extract on Ca47 Absorption in Elderly," *Age and Aging* 1973; 2: 2300-2340.

Wolman, S.L., Anderson, G.H., Marliss, E.B., Jeejeebhoy, K.N., "Zinc total parental nutrition: requirements and metabolic effects," *Gastroenterology* 1979; 76:458-567.

Zen, B.L., *Gynakol* 1998; 110-61.

Step 3C): Reduce Ineffective Organisms in the Body

Balch, J.F. and Balch, P.A., *Prescription for Nutritional Healing,* 2nd Edition, New York: Avery, 1997.

Bergner, P., *The Healing Power of Garlic: The enlightened person's guide of nature's most versatile medicinal plant.* Rocklin, CA: Prima Publishing, 1996.

Berkow, R., *The Merck Manual,* 16th Ed., Rathway, NJ: Merck Research Laboratories, 1992.

Burton Goldberg Group, *Alternative Medicine, The Definitive Guide,* Fife, Washington: Future Medicine Publishing, Inc., 1995.

Carper, J., *The Food Pharmacy,* New York: Bantam Books, 1988.

Chaitow, L., *Amino Acids in Therapy,* Rochester, Vermont: Healing Arts Press, 1988.

Crook, W.G., *The Yeast Connection: A Medical Breakthrough. If You Ever Feel Sick All Over, This Book Could Change Your Life.* New York: Vintage Books, 1986.

Huggins, H.A., *It's All in Your Head: The Link between Mercury Amalgams and Illness,* NY: Avery Publication Group, 1993.

Lininger, S., Wright, J., Austin, S., Brown, D., Gaby, A., *The Natural Pharmacy,* Rocklin, CA: Prima Health, 1998.

Mindell, E., Earl Mindell's Vitamin Bible, New York: Warner Books, 1991.

Rector-Page, L., *How to be Your Own Herbal Pharmacist, An Herbal Formula Reference,* N.G., 1991.

Schmitt, W.H., "Molybdenum for candida albicans patients and other problems," *Digest of Chiropractic Economics* Jan Feb 1991; 56-63.

Stoner, G.D. et al, "The dietary anticancer agent ellagic acid is a potent inhibitor of DNA topoisomerases in vitro," *Nutr Cancer* 1995; 3(2):121-30.

Tierra, M., *The Way of Herbs, With the Latest Developments in Herbal Science,* New York: Pocket Books, 1990.

Truss, O.C., *The Missing Diagnosis,* NY: The Missing Diagnosis Press, 1985.

Step 3D): Replace Enzymes and/or HCL to Aid Digestion, Assimilation and Elimination

Balch, J.F. and Balch, P.A., *Prescription for Nutritional Healing*, 2nd Edition, New York: Avery, 1997.

Burton Goldberg Group, *Alternative Medicine, The Definitive Guide*, Fife, Washington: Future Medicine Publishing, Inc., 1995

Kime, Z.R., *Sunlight* Penryn, CA: World Health Publications, 1980.

Lininger, S., Wright, J., Austin, S., Brown, D., Gaby, A., *The Natural Pharmacy*, Rocklin, CA: Prima Health, 1998.

The Merck Manual, 16th Edition, R Berkow, editor in chief, et al., Rathway, NJ: Merck Research Laboratories, 1992.

Step 3E): Restore Proper Bowel Flora to Optimize Colon Function

Balch, J.F. and Balch, P.A., *Prescription for Nutritional Healing*, 2nd Edition, New York: Avery, 1997.

Burton Goldberg Group, *Alternative Medicine, The Definitive Guide*, Fife, Washington: Future Medicine Publishing, Inc., 1995.

Carper, J., *The Food Pharmacy*, NY: Bantam, 1988; "Yogurt."

Cats, A. et al, "Effect of frequent consumption of a Lactobacillus casei-containing milk drink in Helicobacter pylori-colonized subjects," *Aliment Pharmacol Ther* Feb 2003;17(3):429-35.

Chaitow, L., *Amino Acids in Therapy*, Rochester, Vermont: Healing Arts Press, 1988.

Cutler, E.W., *Winning the War Against Asthma and Allergies, A Drug-Free Cure for Asthma and Allergy Suffers*, Albany, New York: Delmar Publishers, 1998.

Enan, G. et al, "Inhibition of Listeria monocytogenes LMG10470 by plantaricin UG1 in vitro and in beef meat," *Nahrung* Dec 2002;46(6):411-4.

Flynn, S. et al, "Characterization of the genetic locus responsible for the production of ABP-118, a novel bacteriocin produced by the probiotic bacterium Lactobacillus salivarius subsp. salivarius UCC118," *Microbiology* Apr 2002;148(Pt 4):973-84.

Heres, L. et al, "Fermented liquid feed reduces susceptibility of broilers for Salmonella enteritidis," _Poult Sci_ Apr 2003;82(4):603-11.

Hori, T. et al, "Effect of an oral administration of Lactobacillus casei strain Shirota on the natural killer activity of blood mononuclear cells in aged mice," _Biosci Biotechnol Biochem_ Feb 2003;67(2):420-2.

Juarez, Tomas, MS et al, "Influence of pH, temperature and culture media on the growth and bacteriocin production by vaginal Lactobacillus salivarius CRL 1328," _J Appl Microbiol_ 2002;93(4):714-24.

Lininger, S., Wright, J., Austin, S., Brown, D., Gaby, A., _The Natural Pharmacy_, Rocklin, CA: Prima Health, 1998.

Magnusson, J. et al, "Broad and complex antifungal activity among environmental isolates of lactic acid bacteria," _FEMS Microbiol Lett_ Feb 2003 14;219(1):129-3.

Mindell, E., _Earl Mindell's Vitamin Bible_, NY: Warner, 1985.

Payne, S. et al, "In vitro studies on colonization resistance of the human gut microbiota to Candida albicans and the effects of tetracycline and Lactobacillus plantarum LPK," _Curr Issues Intest Microbiol_ Mar 2003;4(1):1-8.

Rodgers, S. et al, "Inhibition of nonproteolytic Clostridium botulinum with lactic acid bacteria and their bacteriocins at refrigeration temperatures," _J Food Prot_ Apr 2003;66(4):674-8.

Sindhu, S.C. and Khetarpaul, N., "Effect of probiotic fermentation on antinutrients and in vitro protein and starch digestibilities of indigenously developed RWGT food mixture," _Nutr Health_ 2002;16(3):173-81.

The Merck Manual, 16th Edition, R Berkow, editor in chief, et al., Rathway, NJ: Merck Research Laboratories, 1992.

Turchet, P. et al, "Effect of fermented milk containing the probiotic Lactobacillus casei DN-114 001 on winter infections in free-living elderly subjects: a randomized, controlled pilot study," _J Nutr Health Aging_ 2003;7(2):75-7.

Step 3: An Addendum: Nutrition: Eat Well to Be Well

Kime Z.R., Sunlight Penryn, CA: World Health Publications, 1980.

Lininger S., Wright J., Austin S., Brown D., Gaby A., The Natural Pharmacy, Rocklin, CA: Prima Health, 1998; "Fish Oil," 160-1.

Passwater R.A., Supernutrition NY: Dial Press, 1975.

Schwarzbein D. and Brown, M., The Schwarzbein Principle II, The Transition, A Regeneration Process to Prevent and Reverse Aging, Deerfield Beach, FL: Health Communications, Inc, 2002.

Schwarzbein D. and Deville, N., The Schwarzbein Principle, The Truth About Losing Weight, Being Healthy and Feeling Younger, Deerfield Beach, FL: Health Communications, Inc, 1999.

Step 4: Reprogram the Body for Allergies/Sensitivities

Balch, J.F. and Balch, P.A., Prescription for Nutritional Healing, 2nd Edition, New York: Avery, 1997.

Burton Goldberg Group, Alternative Medicine, The Definitive Guide, Fife, Washington: Future Medicine Publishing, Inc., 1995.

Cutler, E.W., Winning the War Against Asthma and .... Allergies, A Drug-Free Cure for Asthma and Allergy Sufferers, Albany, NY: Delmar Publishers, 1998: "Allergy Testing," "Genetic and Environmental Causes," "Metabolic Causes," "Chiropractic Misalignments," "Nambudripad Allergy Elimination Technique NAET."

Nambudripad, D.S., Say Good-Bye to Illness, Buena Park, CA: Delta Publishing Co., 1993.

Step 5: Re-Evaluate Emotional Patterns and Remove Limiting Belief Systems

Achterberg, J., Imagery in Healing: Shamanism and Modern Medicine, New York: Random House, 1985.

Bach, E. and Wheeler, F.J., The Bach Flower Remedies, New Canaan, CT: Keats Publishing Co, 1977.

Balch, J.F. and Balch, P.A., Prescription for Nutritional

Healing, 2nd Edition, New York: Avery, 1997.

Barber, T.X., "Physiologic effects of 'hypnotic suggestions'": A critical review of recent research, (1960-64)," Apr 1965; *Psych Bulletin* (63): 201-222.

Black, D., *Healing With Sound*, Springfield, UT: Tapestry Press, 1991.

Burton Goldberg Group, *Alternative Medicine, The Definitive Guide*, Fife, Washington: Future Medicine Publishing, Inc., 1995.

Chopra, D., *Quantum Healing: Exploring the Frontiers of Mind-Body Medicine*, New York: Bantam Books, 1989.

Gilmore, T. et al, eds, *About the Tomatis Method*, Toronto: Listening Center Press, 1989.

Kaslov, L.J., *The Bach Remedies, A Self Help Guide*, New Canaan, CT: Keats Publishing Co, 1977: 3, 9, 22.

Kime, Z.R., *Sunlight*, Penryn, CA: World Health Publications, 1980.

Lininger, S., Wright, J., Austin, S., Brown, D., Gaby, A., *The Natural Pharmacy*, Rocklin, CA: Prima Health, 1998; "Fish Oil," 160-1.

Merritt, S., *Mind, Music, and Imagery*, New York: Plume Press, 1990.

Moyers, B., *Healing and the Mind*, New York: Doubleday, 1993.

Ott, J., *Health and Light*, Old Greenwich, CT: The Devin Adair Co, 1973.

Passwater, R.A., *Supernutrition*, NY: Dial Press, 1975.

Podolsky, E., ed. *Music Therapy*, New York: Philosophical Library, 1954.

Rolf, I., *Rolfing: The Integration of Human Structures*, New York: Harper and Row, 1977.

Schwarzbein, D. and Brown, M., *The Schwarzbein Principle II, The Transition, A Regeneration Process to Prevent and Reverse Aging*, Deerfield Beach, FL: Health Communications, Inc, 2002.

Schwarzbein, D., and Deville, N, *The Schwarzbein Principle, The Truth About Losing Weight, Being Healthy and Feeling Younger*, Deerfield Beach, FL: Health Communications, Inc, 1999.

Selye, H., *Stress without Distress*, New York: Penguin, 1975.

Soilbelman, D., _Industrial and Therapeutic Uses of Music: A Review of the Literature_, New York: Columbia University Press, 1948.

Talbot, M., _The Holographic Universe_, New York: Harper Collins Publishers, 1991.

Walker, M., _The Power of Color: The Art and Science of Making Color Work for You_, Garden City Park, NY: Avery Publishing Group, 1991.

Step 6: Remove Heavy Metals and Other Toxins from the Body

"Indoor Air Pollution, Fact Sheet," American Lung Association, http://www.lungusa.org

"Oral Chelation, The Strongest Natural Treatment for Your Heart, Arteries, Memory and More...," "Qand, A., with Gordon, Garry," _Health and Wellness Update_, Smart Publications 126:1-19, http:\\www.smart-publications.com/ articles/edta-oral-chelation-1. html

"Silicon and Bone Formation," _Nutr Rev_ 1980; 38: 194-195.

"Two Studies Indicate Vitamin D Metabolite Curbs Osteoporosis," _Family Pract News_ March 1984; 15: 2.

Balch, J.F. and Balch, P.A., _Prescription for Nutritional Healing_, 2nd Edition, New York: Avery, 1997.

Biggs, B.L., Melton, L.J., III. "Involutional Osteoporosis," _N Engl J Med_ 1986; 314: 1676-1686.

Brockhaus, A.R. et al. "Intake and health effects of thallium among a population living in the vicinity of a cement plant emitting thallium containing dust," _Int Arch Occup Environ Health_ 1981; 48: 375-389.

Burton Goldberg Group, _Alternative Medicine, The Definitive Guide_, Fife, Washington: Future Medicine Publishing, Inc., 1995.

Chaitow, L., _Amino Acids in Therapy_, Rochester, Vermont: Healing Arts Press, 1988.

Cook, T., _Samuel Hahnemann: The Founder of Homeopathic Medicine_, Wellingborough, Northamptonshire, England: Thorsons, 1981).

Del Giudici, E., Preparata, G., "Superradiance: a new

approach to coherent dynamic behaviors of condensed matter," *Frontier Perspectives* Fall/Winter 1990; 1(2); Philadelphia: Temple University, Frontier Sciences.

Durance, R.A. et al. "Treatment of Osteoporotic Patients. A Trail of Calcium Supplements and Ashed Bone," *Clin. Trials* 1973; 3: 67-73.

Eck, P.C., Wilson, L., *Toxic Metal in Human Health and Disease,* Phoenix, AZ: The Eck Institute of Applied Nutrition and Bioenergetics, Ltd., 1989.

Epstein, O. et al. "Vitamin D, Hydroxyapatite, and Calcium Gluconate in Treatment of Corticol Bone Thinning in Postmenopausal Women With Primary Biliary Cirrhosis," *Am J Clin Nutr* 1982; 36: 426-430.

Faelten, S. et al. *The Complete Book of Minerals for Health,* Emmaus, PA: Rodale Press, 1981.

Follis, R.H. et al. "Studies on copper metabolism XVIII. Skeletal changes associated with copper deficiency in swine," *John Hopkins Hosp Bull* 1955; 97: 405-409.

Frithiof, L. et al. "The relationship between marginal bone loss and serum zinc levels," *Acta Med Scand* 1980; 207: 67-70.

Gaby, A.R. and Wright, J.V., *The Patient's Book of Natural Healing,* Rocklin, CA: Prima Health Book, 1999.

Gallagher, J.C., Riggs, B.L., DeLuca, H.F., "Effect of treatment with synthetic 1:25-dihydroxyVitamin D in postmenopausal osteoporosis," *Clin Res* 1979; 27: 366A.

Gallop, P.M., Lian, J.B/, Hauschka, P.V., "Carboxylated calcium-binding proteins and Vitamin K," *N Eng J Med* 1980; 302: 1460-1466.

Gard, Z.R. and Brown, E.J., "History of Sauna/ Hyperthermia Past and Present Efficacy in Detoxification," *Townsend Letter for Doctors*, June 1992; 470-478, July 1992; 650-660, Oct 1992; 846-854, Aug/Sept 1999; 76-86.

Gerber, R., *Vibrational Medicine,* Santa Fe, NM: Bear and Company, 1988:84.

Hahnemann, S., *Organon of Medicine,* Trans. W. Boericke. New Delhi: B Jain Publishing, 1992.

Heany, R.P., "Thinking Straight About Calcium," *N Eng J Med* 1993; 328(7): 503-505.

Hubbard, L.R., *Clear Body, Clear Mind,* Los Angeles, CA:

Bridge Publications, 1990.

Hunt, C.D., Nielsen, F.H., "Interaction Between Boron and Cholecalciferol in the Chick," in Hawthorne, J.M., Howell, J.M. and White, C.L., eds. *Trace Element Metabolism in Man and Animals*. Berlin, Springer-Verlag, 1982: 597-600.

Johnston, C. et al. "Calcium Supplementation and Increase in Bone Density in Children," *N Eng J Med* 1992; 327: 82-87.

Kilburn, K.H. et al, "Neurobehavioral dysfunction in firemen exposed to polychlorinated biphenyls (PCBs): possible improvement after detoxification," *Arch Environ Health* 1989 Nov-Dec; 44(6): 345-50.

Krop, J., "Chemical sensitivity after intoxication at work with solvents: response to sauna therapy." *J Altern* Complement Med. Spring 1998; 4(1): 77-86.

Lininger, S., Wright, J., Austin, S., Brown, D., Gaby, A., *The Natural Pharmacy*, Rocklin, CA: Prima Health, 1998.

Manzo, L. et al. *Long-term toxicity of thallium in the rat*, Proceed 2nd Int Conf, Clin Chem Mat 1983: 401-405.

McCaslin, F.E., Janes, J.M., "The Effect of Strontium Lactate in the Treatment of Osteoporosis," *Proc Staff Meetings Mayo Clin* 1959; 34: 329-334.

McVicker, M., *Sauna Detoxification Therapy*, McFarland and Co, Box 611, Jefferson, NC 28640, 1997.

Medalle, R., Waterhouse, C., Hahn, T.J., "Vitamin D Resistance in Magnesium Deficiency," *Am J Clin Nutr* 1976; 29: 854-858.

Mills, T.J. et al. "The Use of a Whole Bone Extract in the Treatment of Fractures," *Manitoba Medical Review* 1995; 45: 92-96.

Mindell, E., Earl Mindell's Vitamin Bible, New York: Warner Books, 1991.

Nielsen, E.M. et al. "Microcystalline Hydroxyapatite Compound in Corticosteroid Treated Rheumatoid Patients: A Controlled Study," *Brit Med J* 1978; 2: 1124.

Notoya, K. et al. *Calcif Tissue Int* 1992;51 (1): S3-S6.

Oosterveld et al, "Clinical Effects of Infrared Whole-body Hyperthermia in Patients with Rheumatic Diseases," Departments of Rheumatology and Physiotherapy, Metisch Spectrum Twente and University Twente Enschede, PO Box 50000, 7500 KA Enschede, The Netherlands.

Ozawa, H. et al. *Bone and Mineral* 1992; 19 (1): S21-S26
Pennington, J.A.T. et al. *J Am Diet Assoc*, 86: 1986.

Pfeiffer, C.C., *Zinc and Other Micronutrients,* New Canaan, Connecticut: Keats Publishing, 1978.

Pines, A. et al. "Clinical Trial of MCHC in the Prevention of Osteoporosis Due to Corticosteroid Therapy," *Curr Med Res* 1984; 8(10): 734-742.

Perera, F.P., "Environment and Cancer: Who are Susceptible?" *Science* Nov 7, 1997; 278:1068-73.

Rea, W.J., "Thermal Chamber Depuration and Physical Therapy in Chemical Sensitivity," Volume 4, CRC Press, Boca Raton, 1997; chapter 35: 2433-2479.

Rogers, S., "The Ultimate Solution to Disease," *Total Wellness* May 2000.

Rea, W.J. et al, "Clearing of toxic volatile hydrocarbons from humans," *Bol Assoc Med P R* 1991 July; 83(7):321-4.

Rea, W.J. et al, "Chemical sensitivity in physicians*,"* *Bol Asoc Med P R* 1991 Sept; 83(9): 383-8.

Rector-Page, L., *How to be Your Own Herbal Pharmacist, An Herbal Formula Reference,* N.G., 1991.

Riggs, B.L. et al. "Rates of Bone Loss in the Appendicular and Axial Skeletons of Women," *J Clin Invest* 1986; 7: 1487-1491.

Root, D.E., "Reducing Toxic Body Burdens Advancing in Innovative Technique," *Occupational Health and Safety News Digest* Apr 1986; 2(4).

Schnare, D.W. et al, "Body Burden Reductions of PCB, PBBs and Chlorinated Pesticides in Human Subjects," *Ambio* 1984; 13(5-6): 378-380.

Schnare, D.W. et al, "Evaluation of a Detoxification Regimen for Fat Stored Xenobiotics*,"* *Med Hypoth* 1982; 9:265-82.

Rubik, B., "Frontiers of homeopathic research," *Frontier Perspectives* Spring/Summer 1991; 2(1): Philadelphia: Temple University, Center for Frontier Sciences.

Schmitt, W.H., "Molybdenum for candida albicans patients and other problems," *Digest of Chiropractic Economics* Jan Feb

1991; 56-63.

Schroeder, H.A.. *The Poisons Around Us: Toxic Metals in Food, Air, and Water,* Bloomington, IN: Indiana University Press, 1974.

Smith, R.B., Boericke GW, "Changes caused by succussion on NMR patterns and bioassay of bradykinin triacetate (BKTA) succussion and dilution," *J of the Am Instit of Homeopathy* Nov/Dec 1968; 61: 197-212.

Smith, R.T., Smith, J.C., Fields, M., Reiser, S., "Mechanical Properties of Bone from Copper Deficient Rats Fed Starch or Fructose," *Fed Proc* 1985; 44: 541.

Stellon, A. et al. "Microcystalline Hydroxyapatite Compound in Prevention of Bone Loss In Corticosteroid-Treated Patients With Chronic Active Hepatitis," *Postgrad Med J* 1985; 61: 791-796.

Stepan, J.J. et al. "Prospective Trial of Ossein-Hydroxyapatite Compound in Surgically Induced Postmenopausal Women," *Bone* 1989; 10: 179-185.

Stokinger, H.E., "The metals" in *Patty's Industrial Hygiene and Toxicology,* Vol 2A, Clayton, GD and FE Clayton, eds. New York: John Wiley and Sons, 1981: 1749-1769.

Tierra, M., *The Way of Herbs, With the Latest Developments in Herbal Science,* New York: Pocket Books, 1990.

Vree, T.B. et al, "Excretion of Amphetamines in Human Sweat," *Arch Int Pharmacodyn* 1972; 199: 311-317.

Whitaker, J., *Dr. Whitaker's Guide to Natural Healing*, Prima Publishing, Rockline, CA, 1994: 310-316.

Wilson, T., Katz, J.M., Gray, D.H., "Inhibition of Active Bone Resorption by Copper," *Calcif Tissue Int* 1981; 33:35-39.

Windsor, A.C.M. et al. "The Effect of Whole Bone Extract on Ca47 Absorption in Elderly," *Age and Aging* 1973; 2: 2300-2340.

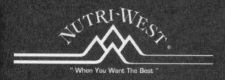
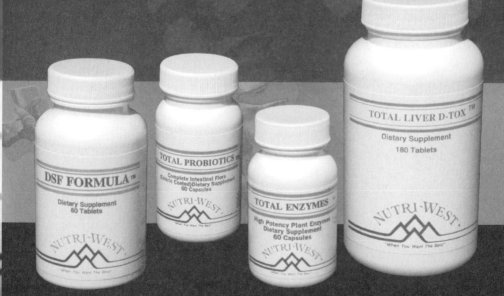

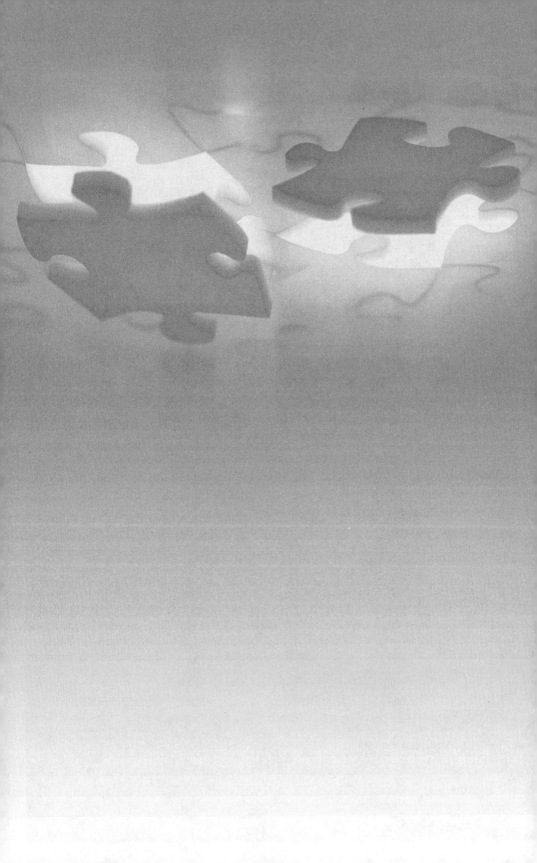

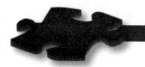

SOLVING THE HEALTH PUZZLE

To find a doctor or practitioner that practices "Dr. Brimhall's 6 Steps to Wellness" protocol, please contact Nutri-West by phone: (800)443-3333 or by e-mail: info@nutri-west.net

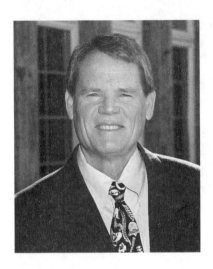

Dr. John Brimhall

Dr. Brimhall has been called "The Father of Wellness Care in Chiropractic." He was lecturing with some of the worlds greatest advocates of health and wellness in the 70's, 80's, 90's and now the 2000's. He is an author, lecturer, formulator of over 70 nutritional products and is also an inventor. He holds patents on two chiropractic instruments. He is a formulator, researcher and consultant for Nutri-West and is a researcher, consultant and inventor for Erchonia Medical.

Dr. Brimhall completed his doctorate in chiropractic from Palmer College of Chiropractic in March of 1971. He was President of the Honor Society and and graduated Cum Laude. He is licensed in Iowa, Arizona and Colorado.

Dr. Brimhall completed his B.A. in Humanities from New Life College of California in 1978. He completed his B.S. in Nutrition from Donsbach University in 1988. He completed his F.I.A.M.A. (Fellow of the International Academy of Medical Acupuncture) in 1988.

Dr. Brimhall is a diplomate of the International College of Applied Kinesiology and member of the American Chiropractic Association.

As an author, Dr. Brimhall has been published on topics of:

- Nutrition in Health & Disease
- Trace Minerals & Toxic Metals
- Manual & Instrument Adjusting Techniques
- Cranial Adjusting
- Visceral Manipulation
- Extremity Adjusting
- Soft Tissue & Myofascial Release Techniques
- Percusson Techniques for Spinal, Extremity & Soft Tissue Treatment
- Rib Adjusting Techniques
- Manual Muscle Testing
- Stress and Emotional Release Techniques
- Allergies and Sensitivities
- Cold Laser Therapy (LLLT)

He has taken Post Graduate work in:

- Motion Palpation
- Gonstead Technique
- E.N.T. by Gibbons
- Activator Methods
- B.E.S.T. by Dr. Morter
- Spinal Biomechanics by Dr. Burl Pettibon
- Applied Kinesiology (Diplomate in ICAK)
- Acupuncture (FIAMA)
- Craniosacral & Visceral Manipulation (Upledger Institute & Dr. Robert Fulford)
- Biocranial Technique by Boyd, DO
- Spinal Rehab
- X-ray

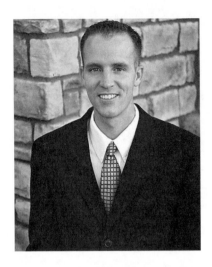

Dr. Brett Brimhall

Dr. Brett Brimhall attended Parker College of Chiropractic in Dallas, TX following his pre-professional courses from Arizona State University. He had achieved proficiency in cranial-sacral and visceral manipulation from the Upledger Institute prior to starting his chiropractic career.

While attending Parker College of Chiropractic he was President of the Percussor, Applied Kinesiology, and Nutrition Clubs. He received his Bachelor of Science in Anatomy and graduated Magna Cum Laude for his Doctorate of Chiropractic degree in December 2000. He was also granted an Outstanding Intern award and the James W. Parker Chiropractic Philosophy Award.

Dr. Brett Brimhall has lectured both nationally and internationally with his father since 1996 on the subject of nutrition, health and wellness. He is currently licensed for Chiropractic, Acupuncture, and Physiotherapy in the state of Arizona where he owns and manages the Brimhall Wellness Center.